C...

nursing

practice

Stoma Care Nursing

Stoma Care Nursing

Catherine Elcoat

SRN, JBCNS (Stoma Care)

Senior Nurse — Stoma Care,
North Tees General Hospital

Baillière Tindall London Philadelphia Toronto
Mexico City Rio de Janeiro Sydney Tokyo Hong Kong

Baillière Tindall   1 St Anne's Road
W.B. Saunders   Eastbourne, East Sussex BN21 3UN, England

West Washington Square
Philadelphia, PA 19105, USA

1 Goldthorne Avenue
Toronto, Ontario M8Z 5T9, Canada

Apartado 26370—Cedro 512
Mexico 4, DF Mexico

Rua Evaristo da Veiga 55, 20° andar
Rio de Janeiro—RJ, Brazil

ABP Australia Ltd, 44–50 Waterloo Road
North Ryde, NSW 2113, Australia

Ichibancho Central Building, 22–1 Ichibancho
Chiyoda-ku, Tokyo 102, Japan

10/fl, Inter-Continental Plaza, 94 Granville Road
Tsim Sha Tsui East, Kowloon, Hong Kong

First published 1986

Typeset by Scribe Design, Gillingham, Kent
Printed and bound in Great Britain by Biddles Ltd, Guildford, Surrey

British Library Cataloguing in Publication Data

Elcoat, Catherine
    Stoma care nursing.—(Current nursing practice)
    1. Gastrointestinal system—Surgery—Nursing—Enterostomy
    I. Title   II. Series
    610.73'677   RD540

ISBN 0 7020 1133 9

Contents

Preface

Research has identified the problems experienced by patients who have undergone surgery resulting in the formation of a faecal or urinary stoma. The recognition of these problems has stimulated an increased interest amongst nurses in stoma care.

Many nurses have little opportunity to develop a high degree of expertise in this field. Some health districts employ trained clinical nurse specialists, equipped to recognize and meet the needs of these patients, whilst in other districts there is still no specialist help available. Thus the service provided varies considerably.

This book aims to satisfy three general objectives:

- Firstly, to equip the generalist nurse with the knowledge she requires to provide a more than adequate standard of care for stoma patients. The text contains basic, practical information pertaining to many aspects of stoma care. This should enable nurses to deal with the variety of problems they encounter in this work.
- Secondly, most of the nursing outlined in the English National Board syllabus for stoma care nursing (Courses 216 and 980) is included. The book should guide all post-registration nurses and others with a special interest in stoma care who are unable to attend a recognized course.
- Thirdly, the book will provide useful information to anyone else involved in the care of stoma patients.

The book is an organized review of the whole topic and should be read completely to give a balanced view of holistic stoma care.

Throughout the text the patient is referred to as 'he' or 'she' as appropriate to the discussion, whilst the nurse assumes the female gender, although of course the authoress recognizes that both patients and nurses may be of either sex.

Catherine Elcoat

Acknowledgements

I would like to express my gratitude to all those people who have in some way influenced the preparation of this book.

Firstly, I wish to acknowledge the help and support I have received from my nursing and medical colleagues at North Tees General Hospital. I am particularly grateful to those consultants who gave up their valuable time to comment on the manuscript and to Dr Edwin Pugh for his constructive criticism and considerable trouble in correcting technicalities in the text.

I would like to thank Mrs Irene Anderson, Stoma Care Secretary, for typing the manuscript into intelligibility; Mrs Elizabeth Clemo, Medical Librarian, for assisting in my literary search; and Mr Ken Watson, Medical Photographer, for providing some of the illustrations included in this book. I am also grateful to Mrs Rosemary Morris, Nursing Editor of Baillière Tindall, and her staff for their advice and guidance.

I must also acknowledge the unknowing contribution of those patients in whose care I have had the privilege to participate. The experience I have gained has undoubtedly influenced my work, as has the exchange of ideas with my fellow stoma care nurses working in the North.

I should like to thank Miss Margaret Best, Director of Nursing Services at North Tees General Hospital, for her continuing professional support, which has been invaluable to me in my role as Clinical Nurse Specialist in Stoma Care.

Lastly, but by no means least, my sincere thanks are due to my husband Richard, without whose unwavering support and encouragement this book could never have been completed.

For Richard

Introduction

Most nurses working in hospital or the community have little opportunity to develop a high degree of expertise in stoma care. They are responsible for many patients and have limited time to spend with those who have a stoma. The stoma care nurse should share her expertise and work as part of the caring team to avoid fragmentation of care; her role should complement rather than detract from the skills of other nurses who are involved with the patient.

The aim of stoma care is to provide a service of management and support both preoperatively and postoperatively for the patient with a stoma and his family and to guide and teach other nurses involved with the patient. This service should supply and maintain a programme of rehabilitation striving to enable the patient to achieve maximum independence and regain a high quality of life.

Although the role of the specialist nurse working in stoma care is exacting, demanding and often stressful, it provides a high degree of job satisfaction. Many nurses are able to continue their support after the patient leaves hospital until he has resumed his previous role in society. A great sense of achievement is gained when the patient is able to demonstrate his ability to enjoy a full and active life once again.

HISTORY OF STOMA CARE NURSING

The earliest documentation of surgically fashioned stomas dates back to the early 1700s. Heister describes the damaged intestine of soldiers injured in battle to the abdominal wall forming an enterostomy. Some of these patients survived.[1] There was, however, no documentation of the specific care of stoma patients in the nursing journals until the late 1930s.[2]

Stoma patients had no access to specialized professional help until the latter half of this century. These unfortunate individuals had to rely upon their improvisational skills and ingenuity, and on advice from each other. In 1949 a small group of stoma patients in Philadelphia, USA formed a self-help group which grew to become the United Ostomy Association. In 1956 the Ileostomy Association of Great Britain and Ireland became the first European group. In 1966 the Colostomy Welfare Group was established, followed in 1971 by the Urostomy Association. These self-help groups offer support and advice to their members on all aspects of living with a stoma.

The first stoma therapist was not a nurse but a patient. Dr R. Turnbull enlisted the help of an ileostomist, Norma Gill, at Cleveland Clinic, Ohio to help with the rehabilitation of new stoma patients in 1958. They went on to establish the first training course for stoma therapists.

Stoma care nursing was pioneered in the UK by Barbara Saunders who was an experienced surgical ward sister at St Bartholomew's Hospital, London and had developed a degree of stoma care expertise. In 1969, together with Ian Todd, a consultant surgeon, she started a monthly clinic for stoma patients.[3] Two other clinics were also operational, one at Birmingham General Hospital organized by Doreen Harris and another at Harold Wood Hospital, Essex, run by Joyce Parsons.[4] Barbara Saunders was subsequently appointed as full-time stoma care nurse in 1971.

Research highlighted a variety of psychological and physical problems encountered by stoma patients.[5,6] Interest in stoma care increased and the patient associations continued to lobby for a better deal for their members. Pressure was brought to bear on appliance manufacturers to improve their products and produce more acceptable appliances and accessories that would improve the quality of life for stoma patients.

In 1978 the DHSS circulated recommendations on the provision of stoma care to all health authorities,[7] and there are now some 200 stoma care nurses in post in Great Britain. The Royal College of Nursing has a stoma care nurses' forum which represents the interests of these nurse specialists and provides a focus for the discussion of problems and exchange of ideas, whilst the World Council of Enterostomal Therapists facilitates the exchange of information internationally.

However, the service available for stoma patients varies considerably between health districts and in some there is still no specialized professional help available. Financial constraint is the familiar excuse when protests are made about these frustrating difficulties,[4] but this may be false economy since an efficient stoma care nurse can provide a much improved service to patients, the cost of which is offset by:

1. Helping to eliminate unnecessarily frequent changes of appliance and thus repeat prescriptions.
2. Diminishing the need for palliative treatment for sore skin.
3. Reducing the number of bed changes.

Clinics and preoperative interviews run by the stoma care nurse can:

1. Reduce stress in the patient and his family.
2. Help reduce the length of hospital stay.
3. Contribute to the more effective use of medical staff time in out patient departments.[7]

In some districts stoma care nurses are being asked to diversify or assume other responsibilities. While this proposal may be economically viable, in some cases it is strongly opposed by many nurses. Such diversification may result in a conflict of interests for the nurse and prove to be a retrograde step for those striving to achieve the status of a clinical specialist.

TRAINING FOR STOMA CARE NURSES

The first specialized training course for stoma care nurses began at St Bartholomew's Hospital, London. Three further training schools have since been established at: North Tees General Hospital, Stockton; Hope Hospital, Salford; and The General Hospital, Birmingham.

The English National Board for Nursing, Midwifery and Health Visiting (ENB) is the statutory body responsible for the course, which was formerly the responsibility of the Joint Board of Clinical Nursing Studies. The aim of the course is to prepare a Registered nurse, who preferably has experience as a sister/charge nurse and has attended a first-line management course, to function as an expert in stoma care nursing.[8]

The course, which takes eight or nine weeks, provides a planned programme of closely integrated theoretical and clinical study. The broad objectives of the outlined curriculum provided by the ENB are: care and management of stoma, communication skills, teaching and research.[9] Based on these broad objectives a planning team then devises specific objectives for a given course.[10] All the training schools offer the same basic course but they are able to utilize additional local facilities and resources.[11] A wide range of topics pertaining to stoma care are included in the programme and particular attention is paid to development of the communication and counselling skills that are essential requisites of a stoma care nurse.

A shortened course of five to eight working days is now available at several centres in the UK for nurses not specializing in stoma care but inevitably coming into contact with patients who have a stoma. The course offers a way of gaining a working knowledge of the basic principles of stoma care and is ideal for Registered or Enrolled nurses working in hospital, community or any other setting whose work involves the nursing of patients with a stoma.[12] However, in no way does this course offer the knowledge and skills essential to equip a nurse to become a clinical specialist in stoma care.

Recently, an advanced course in stoma care has evolved at one centre which it is hoped will become recognized by the English National Board. This course is open to nurses who have completed a recognized eight-week course in stoma care and have been working in the specialty for at least two years. The course lasts for one week and topics such as teaching, counselling and research are studied at a more advanced level. The course also includes discussion of other topics such as transactional analysis, management, clinical budgeting and the law relating to the duty of care.

These courses have resulted in a greater dissemination of knowledge and clinical skills in stoma care to hospital and community nurses.[13]

THE STOMA CARE NURSE

To function efficiently stoma care nurses must have an in-depth knowledge of their specialty and a high degree of clinical competence. Their training should have equipped them with the skills essential to carry out this role, including expertise in counselling and communication, being able to listen actively and express herself clearly. They should be trained in teaching and research methods coupled with the ability to organize an efficient service. A comprehensive knowledge of the resources available locally is also advantageous.

Certain personal attributes are also desirable in nurses endeavouring to fill this exacting role. A stoma care nurse should have a pleasant personality and the ability to get on with others, as well as being approachable, genuine and displaying empathy. They should have a mature outlook with the confidence to 'sell' themselves and the tenacity to carry on their role in the face of opposition. In some situations tact and diplomacy are of paramount importance and the nurse must remain adaptable. A sense of humour coupled with an informal manner and practical common sense is also an advantage. In some clinical settings ingenuity, the ability to improvise and manual dexterity are also essential.

THE ROLE OF THE STOMA CARE NURSE

Stoma care nurses are Registered nurses who have had specialist training in providing a comprehensive service of care and support for patients who have a stoma and their families. They are also a resource within the health district, providing advice and information to any member of the health care team involved in the patient's care. The specific role fulfilled by stoma care nurses varies between health districts but most see patients in the hospital and community as well as holding outpatient stoma care clinics.

To increase the professional credibility of stoma care nursing, the delivery of care must be anchored to research findings. To facilitate this Watson[14] describes a model for stoma care nursing in which she identifies the needs of stoma patients superimposed on fundamental human psychophysiological needs:

- Informational needs.
- Technical stoma management-skill needs.
- Emotional support needs.

Effective stoma care must facilitate these needs being met and the stoma care nurse has several areas of responsibility which include:

- Nursing.
- Teaching.
- Liaison.

- Rehabilitation.
- Record keeping.
- Research.
- Management.

Nursing

The nursing functions of the stoma care nurse must be closely integrated with those of her colleagues, whether working in the hospital ward or in the community. The areas in which her skills are often most valuable are:

- Counselling the patient and his family.
- Providing all the information required by the patient before and after surgery.
- Siting the stoma preoperatively.
- Participating in, and advising on, the care of the stoma and peristomal skin.
- Advising on the choice and use of appliances.
- Visiting the patient after discharge from hospital to provide continuity of care and support.

Teaching

Teaching is of paramount importance if the stoma care nurse is to disseminate her knowledge and improve the care of stoma patients. She may be involved in a variety of teaching situations which include:

- Teaching the patient and his family with regard to caring for and living with a stoma.
- Teaching nurses during their training both in the clinical situation and, more formally, in the classroom.
- Being available to trained nurses to give expert advice as required and keeping nurses in the clinical situation informed of recent developments in stoma care.
- Participating in training sessions for trained nurses and other professionals concerned in the care of stoma patients.
- Participating in symposia both within the health district and for outside agencies if required.

Liaison

Establishing and maintaining effective communication links at all levels is fundamental to an efficient stoma care service. The stoma care nurse liaises with all members of the health care team and other agencies involved in the care and rehabilitation of stoma patients. She can act as a link between the patient and other resources that may help to enable him to resume his previous lifestyle. The stoma care nurse can help to facilitate a smooth transition for the patient between hospital and home by liaising with ward and community nursing staff.

Rehabilitation

One of the primary aims of stoma care nursing is to help the stoma patient achieve full rehabilitation. The stoma care nurse is involved in encouraging the patient to resume his interests and hobbies. She may be involved with the occupational health department at his work place or she may enlist the help of other experts to organize retraining. The stoma care nurse endeavours to ensure that every possible action is taken to enable the patient to resume a full and undiminished role in society as soon as possible.

Record keeping

The stoma care nurse must ensure that accurate records are maintained on all patients treated. She should endeavour to keep up-to-date information on all patients within her health district who have a stoma. A record of her own daily activities, such as number of patients seen in various settings, is also advantageous. Provided these accurate records are available a colleague could maintain the service if the nurse were absent for any reason. The records are also most useful if the nurse specialist is called upon to justify her existence, particularly in these days of stringent financial constraint. Many stoma care nurses set aside a specific time each day to spend in their office on clerical work. If this time is known to other team members and patients it can be a useful contact arrangement and may reduce interruptions made at other times when the nurse is concentrating on specific patients.

The problem-solving approach of the nursing process is ideal for stoma care nursing. The nurse who is endeavouring to provide the very highest standards of care often recognizes that this approach represents a logical and systematic method of taking a holistic view of the patient and achieving her aims.

Research

Nursing practice today should be based on research, and in fact stoma care nurses are often involved in research and frequently write articles for the nursing press to further the knowledge base of their specialty. Their contribution to research may include:

- Providing data for research projects.
- Participating in clinical trials of products and equipment.
- Undertaking a research project to improve patient care.
- Keeping abreast of new developments and techniques in stoma care.

Management

In many health districts the stoma care nurse works with a high degree of autonomy. She often has managerial responsibility for the stoma care service and works as an independent practitioner. She may be a budget holder and is often responsible for the ordering and maintenance of stoma care stocks. There is a move in the NHS that aims to make the user in the clinical situation more responsible for budgeting. This may involve the stoma care nurse in both working in a cost-effective manner and providing accurate data of her activities for each clinician's patients so that the cost of service can be 're-charged' accordingly.

RESOURCES REQUIRED FOR A STOMA CARE SERVICE

To function efficiently the stoma care nurse must have certain resources available. A room in which to counsel patients in privacy is essential, preferably a room that creates an informal atmosphere with comfortable chairs for the counsellor and client of a similar height with no barrier (such as a desk) between. With careful thought and planning this room can double as an office. A clinical area with a couch, running water, mirror and good light is also required to enable the nurse to carry out practical stoma care procedures. It is desirable if these facilities are within a conventional outpatient department so that no stigma is associated with sitting in the waiting area. The stoma care nurse should also have access to medical advice; to facilitate this many clinics run concurrently with a surgical clinic. It is vital that clinics are easily accessible to those who need to attend. For this reason, hospitals and health centres which usually have a regular transport service are generally most suitable.

To be able to offer patients a choice of appliance the stoma care nurse should have at her disposal a comprehensive range of products. This will also enable the nurse to select the product most likely to suit the needs of an individual with a specific problem. Access to clerical help is needed as the stoma care nurse is required to correspond with other members of the health care team regarding specific patients. A secretary may also take messages when the nurse is unavailable. However, she must never act as a barrier preventing the patient gaining access to the nurse.

Carrying a 'bleep' enables the stoma care nurse to be contacted direct at most times, and paging devices that have a range of several miles are available. Some centres provide a 24-hour on-call service which gives patients and other professionals access to stoma care expertise at all times. They feel it is essential to maintain a continuous level of cover.[15] Obviously for this arrangement to be practical at least three nurses interested and skilled in the specialty must agree to participate. Calls are not usually a common occurrence if well-planned care and visits are executed within normal working hours. However, it is often reassuring to patients to know that help and advice is always available. This arrangement also facilitates the preoperative siting of stomas created for patients in an emergency situation. The nurse who visits patients in their own homes will require transport and a mileage allowance is usually paid. The stoma care nurse should also have practical support from at least one other nurse with stoma care expertise who can then provide relief during holidays or illness. It is important, however, that the two also work together regularly to ensure that there is continuity of care and the helper is kept up to date with current practice.

The nursing process and individualized patient care is breaking down the traditional defences of a task-orientated environment.[16] This approach to nursing enables the nurse to become closer to her patient emotionally, which may result in increased stress. Stoma care nurses undertake counselling regularly, which is also stressful since they open themselves to the patient's pain. A long-term relationship is usually developed with the patients and she becomes closely involved in their lives. Therefore, it is essential that the stoma care nurse herself has access to emotional support from either her nurse manager or her peer group. These support sessions should occur on a regular basis so that issues can be shared and discussed openly, rather than waiting until a crisis arises. Regular contact with other nurses working in the specialty is also advantageous.

Many patients cannot differentiate between different nurse grades thus all may be type-cast as too busy to have time to talk. As the aim of stoma care nursing is to develop a close relationship with the patient facilitating counselling and emotional support, many stoma care nurses do not wear uniform because this may create a barrier. Uniform is often not appropriate when visiting in the community as the patient may not wish neighbours to know he has a stoma, and regular visits may provoke embarrassing questions. If the nurse does not wear a uniform she may receive a small clothing allowance.

The provision of a stoma care service requires a considerable financial commitment from the health authority. However, much of this expense may be recouped as previously discussed. There is evidence that many patients experience difficulties in coping with their stoma and suffer considerable psychological distress.[5,6] However, more research is required to evaluate the impact that stoma care nurses have had upon the rehabilitation of stoma patients.[17] It is hoped that by providing an individually tailored programme of help and support for these patients the stoma care nurse is effective in overcoming problems, facilitating rehabilitation and improving the quality of life enjoyed by these individuals.

REFERENCES

1. Richardson, R.G. (1973) *The Abominable Stoma: A Historical Survey of the Artificial Anus.* Abbott Laboratories.
2. Plumley, S. (1939) Care of ileostomy. *American Journal of Nursing*, **39**, 275.
3. Saunders, H.B. (1974) Stoma care nurse: a new role. *Nursing Times*, 578–579.

4. Brady, N. (1984) A history of caring. *Senior Nurse*, *23* (5 September), 8–10.
5. Devlin, H.B., Plant, J.A. & Griffin, M. (1971) The aftermath of surgery for ano-rectal cancer. *British Medical Journal, 3*, 413–418.
6. Biermann, H.J. (1966) Statistical survey of problems in patients with colostomy and ileostomy. *American Journal of Surgery*, *112*, 647–650.
7. Health Services Development (1978) *The Provision of Stoma Care*. DHSS publication HC78, London.
8. Finn, B. (1974) Training the stoma care nurse. *Nursing Times*, 18 April, 579.
9. Outline Curriculum in Stoma Care Nursing for State Registered Nurses: Course 216. London Joint Board of Clinical Nursing Studies.
10. Brady, N. (1982) Training nurses in stoma care. *Stoma Care News, No. 1*, December, p. 6.
11. Gardner, J. (1985) Stoma care nurses. In *Stoma Care To-day*.Ed. Devlin, H.B. Oxford: The Medicine Publishing Foundation. p.44–45.
12. Editorial (1983) Ideal course for nurses and midwives. *Stoma Care News*, *4*, November, p. 9.
13. Breckman, B. (1982) Stoma nursing in the 1990s. *Nursing Times*, 24 February, p. 326–328.
14. Watson, P.G. (1985) Meeting the needs of patients undergoing ostomy surgery. *Journal of Enterostomal Therapy, 12*, 121–124.
15. Dellipiani, A.W. & Plant, J.A. (1978) Organisational aspects and the continuity of psychological and social care of patients. In *Intestinal Stomas*, Ed. Todd, I.P., Chap. 18, pp. 154–162. London: Heinemann.
16. Dowd, D. & Martin, T. (1984) Oasis on Mondays. *Nursing Times*, 17 October, p. 50–51.
17. Devlin, H.B. (1985) Second opinion. *Health and Social Services Journal*, 17 January, p. 82.

1   Anatomy and physiology associated with stoma care

When considering anatomy and physiology in relation to stoma care it is not only essential to consider the gastrointestinal tract and bowel function but also the male and female genitourinary systems and the skin.

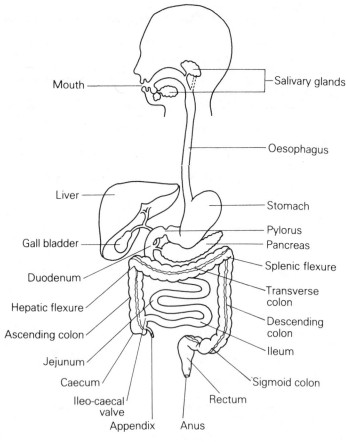

Fig. 1. *The alimentary tract.*

THE ALIMENTARY TRACT

The alimentary tract stretches from the mouth to the anus and in the adult is some seven metres in length. It stores food in the stomach and then converts it to assimilable small molecules in the intestine. Undigestible material is then stored in the colon until it can be conveniently eliminated through the rectum and anus.

The tract is basically a tube of varying diameters made up of four main layers:

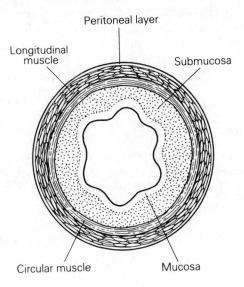

Fig. 2. *Cross-section of alimentary tract.*

Mucosa

The mucosa lines the tract and is made up of epithelial cells and secretory glands. The surface area can be expanded by the thin muscle layer, the muscularis mucosae. It has a good supply of blood and lymphatic vessels and is both absorptive and secretory.

Submucosa

This is a layer of connective tissue joining the mucosa to the muscular layers. There is a network of nerve endings, the submucosal plexus.

Muscle

The mouth and upper pharynx have a striated (voluntary) muscle layer which is arranged in complex sheets to allow mastication and swallowing. A smooth muscle layer surrounds the oesophagus, stomach, and the small and large intestine. This muscle is not under voluntary control and, therefore, moves repeatedly whether the person is awake or asleep.

The smooth muscle is arranged in two sheets, a circular inner sheet and a longitudinal outer sheet. It is controlled by autonomic nerves and is responsible for the propulsive waves that transport food substances along the tract—peristalsis.

The lower 5 cm or so of the large bowel are surrounded by a cuff, a sphincter of striated muscle which is under full voluntary control. This sphincter maintains continence and allows the passage of flatus and faeces at will.

Peritoneum

This is a layer of strong connective tissue. The peritoneum covers most of the gastrointestinal tract in the abdomen. The oesophagus in the chest does not have this layer nor does the large bowel in the pelvis.

FUNCTION OF THE ALIMENTARY TRACT

Mouth

Functions

1. Mastication of the food by the teeth.
2. Mixing the food with saliva.

Oesophagus

Functions

1. Waves of contraction convey food bolus to the cardiac sphincter of the stomach.
2. The sphincter at the lower end of the oesophagus relaxes and food enters the stomach.

Stomach

Functions

1. A reservoir for food.
2. Mixing of food with gastric juice to form chyme.
3. Production of gastric juice, which is acidic (pH 1.5–3.5).
4. Absorption of water, some drugs and alcohol.
5. Control of output of food into the duodenum.
6. Secretion of intrinsic factor.

Small intestine

The small intestine is made up of three parts:

1. Duodenum.
2. Jejunum.
3. Ileum.

During the journey along the small intestine digestion of the food is completed and almost all the nutrients and much of the water are absorbed.

Duodenum

Functions

1. Reception of pancreatic juice and bile from the outlet to the common bile duct, both of which are alkaline (pH 7.8–8.0).
2. Major role in digestion of protein, fats and starch; the food is mixed with pancreatic juice and bile.
3. Absorption of calcium, iron and magnesium.

Jejunum and ileum

In this part of the small intestine the mucosa is folded into valvulae conniventes and covered with about 5 000 000 projections called villi. The surface of each villus is covered in about 1000 microvilli, forming a brush border. This arrangement is said to increase the surface area for absorption by about 600 times. Each villus has a blood supply via a capillary network and a branch of the lymphatic system called a lacteal. Blood supply and cell activity increase after meals.

Functions
1. Mixing of partially digested food with intestinal juice.
2. Completion of digestion of fat, protein and carbohydrate.
3. The main site for the absorption of foods, as follows:

- *Carbohydrates:* These are mainly absorbed in the jejunum where they cross the mucosal surface of the villi to enter the capillary network of the portal circulation.
- *Proteins:* These enter the capillary network in the villi to the portal circulation.
- *Fats:* These enter the lacteal as chyle and drain into the lymphatic circulation and then, eventually, into the venous circulation via the thoracic duct. However, 10–20% may be absorbed directly into the portal circulation.
- *Water and electrolytes:* Sodium, chloride, calcium, iron, potassium, magnesium, phosphate and bicarbonate are absorbed here. Some water is absorbed by osmosis provided the contents of the intestine are hypotonic. If they are hypotonic water will be attracted into the gut from the bloodstream.
- *Vitamins:* Fat and water soluble vitamins are absorbed in the terminal ileum. Vitamin B_{12} is also absorbed in the terminal ileum after it has combined with intrinsic factor from the stomach.
- *Bile salts:* These are reabsorbed in the terminal ileum as part of the enterohepatic circulation.

The large intestine

The large intestine is about 1.5 m long; it has no villi but its lumen is wider than that of the small intestine providing the capacity to store food residue. Movement is much slower. The longitudinal muscle bonds are incomplete and are gathered into bands called taeniae coli; between the taenia the colon pouches into the haustra, giving it a sacculated effect.

Functions
1. Absorption of water; the amount depends upon the time the residue remains in the colon—the greater the time, the more water is absorbed.

2. Absorption of sodium to the portal circulation.
3. Secretion of mucus, which gives the colonic contents an alkaline nature—pH 8.
4. Bacteria live in the colon naturally, e.g. bacteroides, streptococci and lactobacilli. These produce Vitamin K, thiamine and riboflavin in small amounts.
5. Absorption of drugs such as analgesics and steroids which may be administered rectally.
6. Storage of faeces until defecation is appropriate.

BOWEL FUNCTION

Normal defecation

Faeces are made up of 75% water and 25% solid constituents. These are undigested foodstuffs (particularly cellulose), dead epithelial cells, bacteria, mucus, bile pigments (stercobilin) and small amounts of sodium and potassium. Two substances—indole and skatole—which arise from bacterial decomposition give faeces its characteristic odour. On average, those eating a Western diet eliminate 100–150 g of faeces daily. Those from cultures where the diet includes a high proportion of fibre may pass considerably more. The average person will defecate five to seven times weekly[2] but bowel habit is very much an individual phenomenon.

The gastrocolic reflex occurs usually after meals, particularly in the morning. The reflex causes the terminal ileum to contract and fluid faeces are allowed to enter the caecum. Similarly 'mass movement' occurs within the colon propelling bowel contents towards the rectum. The rectum is usually empty until just prior to defecation. When faeces fill the rectum the walls are distended and the urge to defecate is felt. This may be referred to as a 'call to stool' and gives rise to afferent impulses passing to the sacral spinal cord.

The internal anal sphincter is made of smooth muscle and is controlled by the autonomic nervous system. Therefore it is not under conscious control. The sacral parasympathetic fibres cause the sphincter to relax while the sympathetic fibres cause constriction. The external anal sphincter is composed of striated muscle and is under voluntary control. If it is inconvenient to defecate the stimulus can be overcome by contraction of the external sphincters; the sensation passes after a few moments and does not normally return for several hours. When defecation occurs the internal and external sphincters open, the intra-abdominal pressure is increased by lowering the diaphragm and contracting the abdominal muscles. The muscles of the pelvic floor and the rectum also contract and the faeces are expelled.

The transit time between the ingestion of food and subsequent defecation is very variable and depends on physical, physiological and psychological factors.[2,3] The average is around 24 hours but one study revealed that in elderly patients in hospital it may be as long as three weeks.[4]

Flatus

There are three possible sources of gas within the gut:

- Ingested air.
- Gas produced chemically within the gut.
- Diffusion from the blood.[5]

The largest proportion of colonic gas is produced by bacterial fermentation. Flatus consists of nitrogen, carbon dioxide, hydrogen, methane and hydrogen sulphide; the amount produced varies between individuals and may be about 500 ml in 24 hours. The constituents of the diet also influence the amount of flatus produced. The characteristic obnoxious odour can be attributed to hydrogen sulphide and skatole.

Implications for stoma patients

The absence of the peritoneum in the lower pelvis makes the lower rectum relatively delicate and adds to the difficulties of surgical anastomoses at this site. Low pelvic anastomoses are prone to leak, leading to sepsis and fistula, so a temporary stoma may have to be created. (See Chapter 3.) Patients who have a stoma do not defecate via the rectum and thus do not have the advantage of anal sphincter muscles. They are, therefore, rendered incontinent. Flatus is also passed via the stoma and thus the patient has no control over its emission.

Ileostomy patients

Most patients who have an ileostomy have had the colon removed. Thus they lose some of their ability to reabsorb water in their faeces, which is excreted together with sodium from the ileostomy. A well-functioning ileostomy may excrete 60 mmol of sodium and 500 ml of water each day; this is two to three times the amount normally found in faeces.[6] The body compensates for this by diminishing the urinary output or adjusting to a new balance. The way in which the body adapts after ileostomy is not fully understood. However, some physiological adaptation must occur as it is recognized that about 1500 ml of fluid faeces enter the colon at the caecum[7] whilst surveys have shown average ileostomy output to be 500–600 ml per day.[6,8] Increased output of antidiuretic hormone,[9] increased output of aldosterone[8] and increase in the size of small bowel villi[10] are possible explanations. Some patients pass far greater volumes than this, depleting the body of fluid and salts.

If part of the ileum has also been removed the patient may have difficulty with absorption of nutrients and vitamins. The terminal ileum reabsorbs bile salts and its removal can result in an increased incidence of gall stone formation. Vitamin B_{12} is also absorbed in the terminal ileum and failure to absorb this vitamin will result in pernicious anaemia two to three years after surgery when stores maintained in the liver are depleted. Effluent from the ileum is not only fluid but also strongly alkaline and may contain proteolytic enzymes. Thus contact with the peristomal skin can very quickly produce excoriation. The ileum, which is normally sterile, may also become colonized with bacteria from outside the body.

If the surgeon creates a reservoir for faecal waste using the ileum, (e.g. Koch reservoir or Parks Pouch) the patient may have problems with reabsorption of waste through the reservoir as the ileum does not lose its reabsorptive qualities (see Chapter 2). This may also be the case if a piece of the ileum is used as a conduit to divert urine.

Colostomy patients

The position of the colostomy in the colon will determine the amount of water lost in the faeces. The sigmoid colon is important in controlling the consistency of faeces,[3] thus a transverse colostomy will emit a semi-fluid stool whilst a colostomy created from the sigmoid colon may well emit formed faeces.

The effects of flatus, diarrhoea and constipation may be much more traumatic to patients with a colostomy than those with unaltered bowel anatomy and may be more difficult to treat. The characteristic odour of faeces and flatus may be a constant worry as the patients have no control over their emission. It is therefore imperative that they are fitted with a suitable odourproof appliance in which they can have confidence.

THE URINARY SYSTEM

The urinary system consists of the kidneys, ureters, bladder and urethra.

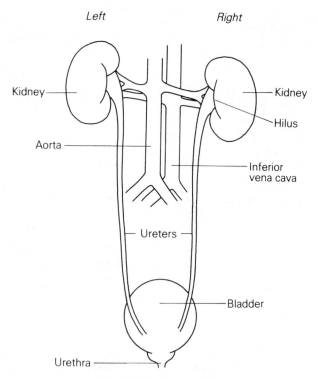

Fig. 3. *The urinary system.*

Urine is formed in the kidney, which consists of about 1 000 000 nephrons. Urine is produced by three processes:

1. Filtration under pressure through the glomerulus of the nephron.
2. Selective reabsorption in the kidney tubule of water, glucose, salts and ions which the body requires. Most of the water and salts are reabsorbed.
3. Active secretion by the cells of the kidney tubule of certain waste substances in the blood such as urea.

Reabsorption of water is controlled by the secretion of antidiuretic hormone (ADH) from the posterior lobe of the pituitary gland. A decrease in the secretion of ADH results in less water being reabsorbed and a larger volume of urine being produced. An average individual passes approximately 1.5 litres of urine daily. Normally urine has a pH of 7.4 and a specific gravity of 1015–1025. Its constituents are water, salts and protein waste products, i.e. urea, uric acid and creatinine, in the following proportions:

Water 96%
Urea 2%
Uric acid and salts 2%.

The ureters carry urine from the kidney to the bladder. They are about 25–30 cm long and approximately 3 mm in diameter, passing from the renal pelvis to the ureteric orifices of the bladder.

The bladder is a reservoir for urine. When empty it lies wholly within the pelvis but as it fills with urine it distends and expands upwards and forwards into the abdominal cavity. The bladder can hold over 500 ml of urine but at this size it is painful, the desire to micturate usually being felt when the bladder contains 250–300 ml of urine.

The urethra in the male is 18–20 cm long and serves as a canal for both the urinary and reproductive systems, conveying urine and seminal fluid. In the female it is approximately 4 cm long and serves only the urinary system. There are internal and external sphincters to the urethra: the internal sphincter is involuntary and the external sphincter is under voluntary control.

Micturition

Urine constantly passes into the bladder from the ureters; when there is between 200 and 300 ml of urine in the bladder there is an increase in tension which stimulates sensory nerves, initiating the desire to micturate. As these impulses increase the motor impulses cause a reflex contraction of the bladder and relaxation of the internal sphincter. The external sphincter is under the control of the pudendal nerve. Once the skill of inhibiting the spinal reflex is learned micturition can be controlled.

Implications for stoma patients

Following urinary diversion

Diversion of the urinary flow away from the bladder eliminates the reservoir, so urine is voided constantly via the stoma. The indications for urinary diversion and the alternative procedures are discussed in Chapters 2 and 3. The patient has no control of micturition following urinary diversion as urinary continence is dependent upon the function of the bladder sphincters. Excision of the bladder has little effect on bowel function.

Following rectal excision

Abdominoperineal excision of the rectum can result in some disruption in the function of the bladder and urinary tract. Moreover this operation is most commonly performed in those over 60 years of age and there may be some pre-existing urinary dysfunction, in the female due to lack of oestrogen or in the male due to an enlarged prostate.

Following removal of the rectum the bladder may fall backwards, as support is compromised. Prolapse and sphincter insufficiency in the female may also increase. If the levator ani muscle which forms the pelvic floor is removed this can result in bladder dysfunction and urinary retention. Damage to the nerves innervating the bladder and urethra will impair sensation and inhibit the action of the bladder. The bladder may then tend to overfill, stretching the deltrusor muscle, rendering it less efficient and unable to contract adequately. This in turn may impair the emptying of the bladder resulting in stagnation of urine and possible infection and inflammatory changes which further increase dysfunction. This process may be worse in the male if there is prostatic enlargement.

Impaired continence may also result after excision of the rectum, partly due to the infection causing an irritation resulting in uninhibited bladder contractions. Another possible cause of postoperative incontinence is damage to the pelvic nerves which innervate the bladder and sphincter controlling the tone of the urethra, keeping it closed. If this tone is compromised the patient will be incontinent when the pressure in the bladder rises. The effects of pelvic nerve damage on sexual function are discussed later in this chapter.

MALE GENITAL ORGANS

The male genital organs are situated both internally in the pelvis and external to the body. The internal organs lie in close proximity to the bladder and rectum.

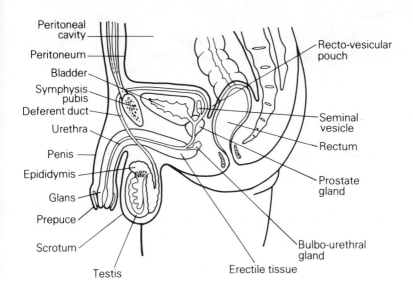

Fig. 4. *The male pelvic organs.*

The physiology of sexual function in the male is not totally understood but a sequence of events is indicated.[11] Satisfactory male sexual function involves four co-ordinated processes—erection, emission, ejaculation and detumescence—and is dependent on an intact autonomic nervous system.[12]

Erection

The penis becomes erect when the erectile tissue (corpora cavernosa) becomes engorged with blood. Erection may result from psychological stimulus such as visual images or erotic thoughts (psychogenic erection); this occurs via the thoracolumbar sympathetic nerves and the sacral parasympathetic nerve fibres. Local tactile stimulation of the penis instigates reflexogenic erection initiated by afferent fibres in the pudendal nerves and efferent fibres in the nervi erigentes. The nerves that control penile erection form the hypogastric plexus which lies in the fat in the side wall of the rectum.

Emission

Emission is the first stage of ejaculation during which the smooth muscle of the epididymus, vasa deferentia, seminal vesicles and prostatic capsule contracts and semen enters the posterior urethra. Emission is primarily controlled by the sympathetic nervous system.

Ejaculation

During ejaculation the seminal fluid is transported along the urethra and expelled from the body. This occurs when the bladder neck closes and parasympathetic nerve stimulation causes rhythmic contraction of the striated ischiocavernosus and bulbocavernosus muscle. This process is usually associated with a release of built-up body tension and intense pleasure—orgasm. It should, however, be noted that the male may experience orgasm without ejaculation or erection occurring and ejaculation may occur without the penis being erect.[13]

Detumescence

During this phase the genitalia return to the pre-excitory state. Once autonomic, sensory and motor stimuli cease, blood is expelled from the engorged penis which resumes its flaccid state.

Implications for stoma patients

If the hypogastric plexus is damaged during surgery to remove the rectum then impairment of sexual function (both erection and ejaculation) will result due to absence of both sympathetic and parasympathetic nervous stimulation. Sexual function is usually also impaired following cystectomy. (Other sexual implications are discussed in Chapter 16.)

In the male the bladder lies in close proximity to the rectum, so surgery to one may involve the other. Disease or infection may result in fistula formation between bowel and bladder (colovesicle fistula) which may require formation of stoma to divert the flow.

FEMALE GENITAL ORGANS

The internal female genital organs (the ovaries, fallopian tubes, uterus and vagina) are situated in the lesser pelvis.

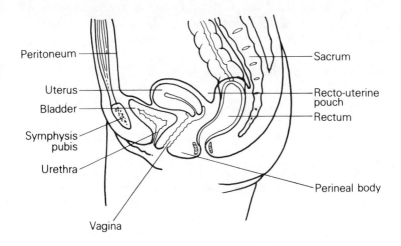

Fig. 5. *The female pelvic organs.*

The specific physiology of menstruation and reproduction is quite complex. However, there are some pertinent considerations when discussing stoma care and the possible implications of creating a stoma in the female patient.

Implications for stoma patients

The rectum, vagina and bladder lie in close proximity in the female pelvis, thus surgery to one organ may involve the others. Colonic disease (e.g. Crohn's disease or severe pelvic sepsis) can result in fistula formation from one organ to another, i.e. rectovaginal fistula. In this case faeces or urine may be discharged via the vagina. This may require the formation of a stoma to divert the flow.

Following rectal excision a raw area is left, in many cases the uterus falls back into the space vacated by the rectum and becomes stuck to the posterior pelvic wall; this alters the angle of the vagina and may result in dyspareunia, particularly if intercourse is attempted in certain positions. The ovaries may prolapse into the pouch of Douglas after surgery, which can result in pain if they are compressed during intercourse. If there has been pelvic infection due to disease or abscess formation the fallopian tubes may be involved, leading to infertility as a result of the tubes becoming blocked. A decrease in blood supply to the vagina and external genitalia may result in a lack of lubrication by secretions from the vaginal and cervical glands, resulting in dyspareunia.

Other considerations such as sexual problems, pregnancy and contraception are discussed in Chapter 16.

THE SKIN

The skin consists of two layers, the outer horny layer called the *epidermis* and a lower layer called the *dermis*.

The skin is normally an effective resilient barrier covering the body and protecting deeper tissue. The epidermis is non-vascular and consists of stratified epithelium. It has two zones, the horny zone and the germinative zone. The horny zone has three layers:

1. *The stratum corneum:* This is the outer layer and the cells are flat without a nucleus, the protoplasm having become

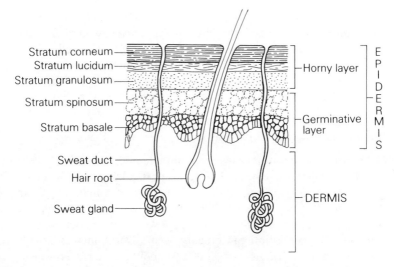

Fig. 6. *The layers of the skin.*

keratin, which is waterproof. The epidermal cells which synthesize keratin are known as keratinocytes and they originate in the basal layer of the epidermis.

2. *The stratum lucidum:* This is made up of cells with clear protoplasm. Some have nuclei which are flat.
3. *The stratum granulosum:* This consists of several layers of cells with nuclei and a protoplasm that is granular.

The deeper germinative zone has two layers:

4. *The stratum spinosum.*
5. *The stratum basale.*

Cells originate in the stratum basale where they are known as basal cells. They then grow up into the stratum spinosum where they are known as prickle cells. When the cells reach the stratum granulosum they are known as granular cells, prior to becoming a keratinocyte in the outer stratum corneum. This ascent through the living layers of the skin takes about 15 days. After losing their nucleus the cells then remain on the stratum corneum for about a further 15 days.

The dermis is a fibroelastic bed which supports and nourishes the epidermis and its appendages. The stratum corneum is resistant to quite strong acids but is more vulnerable to alkaline substances. It can exclude harmful chemicals whilst allowing topical allergens and treatments to be admitted. The cells of the stratum corneum affect the rate at which molecules can pass through to the deeper layers. The speed of this movement is increased if the temperature or humidity of the skin is raised.

Implications for stoma patients

The skin around a stoma is very vulnerable and if it once becomes damaged it can prove difficult to treat, particularly with the added problem of affixing an adhesive appliance. Exudate from an ileostomy is often strongly alkaline and may still contain the proteolytic enzymes of digestion. If allowed into contact with the skin severe excoriation can quickly occur. Keratinocytes usually remain on the stratum corneum for about 15 days. However, removal of an adhesive appliance will pull off a layer of cells each time it is changed. If this changing is too frequent damage to the skin will ensue.

As previously stated the passage of molecules through the skin occurs at a faster rate if the temperature or humidity is increased. If the adhesive layer of an appliance prevents normal function of the skin the temperature and humidity may rise and the speed at which irritant substances are absorbed will be increased. This can result in skin irritation.

REFERENCES

1. Hinchcliffe, S.M. (1981) The normal function of the alimentary tract. In *Stoma care*. Ed. Breckman, B., Chap 2, pp. 16–51. Beaconsfield: Beaconsfield.
2. Thompson, M. & Bottomley, H. (1980) Normal and abnormal bowel function. *Nursing, 17*, (September) 721–722.
3. Brooks, S.L. (1984) Disturbances of bowel function. *Nursing, 30*, (October) 870–876.
4. Brocklehurst, J.C. & Yunis Khan, M. (1969) A study of faecal stasis in old age and the use of Dorbanex in its prevention. *Gerontology Clinics, II*, 293–300.
5. Eastham, E.J. (1983) Wind. *Update*, 15 February, 531–542.
6. Hill, G.L. (1982) Metabolic complications of ileostomy. *Clinics in Gastroenterology, 11*, 16 May, pp. 260–267.
7. Debongnie, J.C. & Phillips, S.F. (1978) Capacity of the human colon to absorb fluid. *Gastroenterology, 74*, 698–703.
8. Kennedy, H.J., Al-Dujaili, E.A.S., Edwards, C.R.W., Truelove, S.C. (1983) Water and electrolyte balance in subjects with permanent ileostomy. *Gut, 24*, 702–705

9. La Veen, H.H., Lyons, A. & Becker, E. (1962) Physiological adaptation to ileostomy. *American Journal of Surgery*, *103*, 35–43.
10. Wright, H.K., Cleveland, J.C., Tilson, M.D. & Herskovic, T. (1969) Morphology and absorptive capacity of the ileum after ileostomy in man. *American Journal of Surgery, 177*, 242–245.
11. Young, C.H. (1982) Sexual implications of stoma surgery, Part I. *Clinics in Gastro-enterology*, May *11, No. 2*, pp 383–391.
12. Gaum, L.D. (1982) Neurological sequelae of abdominoperineal resection. *Surgical Clinics of North America, 62*, 1075–1083.
13. Shipes, E.A. & Lehr, S.T. (1980) *Sexual Counselling for Ostomates*, Vol. 1, Springfield, Ill.: C.C. Thomas. pp. 3–18.

2 Conditions that may require surgery involving a stoma

Stomas may be divided into three classifications: input stomas; diverting stomas; and output stomas.

1. *Input stomas:* These are usually temporary and facilitate nutrients being put into the gut, e.g. gastrostomy, jejunostomy.
2. *Diverting stomas:* These divert the contents of the gastrointestinal tract away from diseased or damaged gut, e.g. loop ileostomy, loop colostomy.
3. *Output stomas:* These provide an outlet for the elimination of body waste, usually following excision of an excretory organ, i.e. bladder or bowel, e.g. 'iliac' colostomy, ileostomy, ileal conduit.

There are a variety of conditions which may predispose to surgery involving the creation of a stoma. The most common conditions are described in this chapter.

CONDITIONS INVOLVING THE COLON

- Ulcerative colitis.
- Crohn's disease.
- Familial polyposis coli.
- Carcinoma.
- Diverticular disease.
- Colonic obstruction.
- Bowel ischaemia.
- Anorectal incontinence.
- Trauma.
- Irradiation damage.

CONDITIONS INVOLVING THE URINARY SYSTEM

- Bladder cancer.
- Contracted bladder.
- Urinary incontinence.
- Failed uretero-colic anastomosis.

PAEDIATRIC CONDITIONS

Congenital abnormalities

- Anorectal anomalies.
- Bladder exstrophy.
- Cloacal exstrophy.
- Spina bifida.
- Hirschsprung's disease.
- Necrotizing enterocolitis.
- Meconium ileus.
- Trauma.

INFLAMMATORY BOWEL DISEASES THAT MAY REQUIRE SURGERY INVOLVING A STOMA

Ulcerative colitis

'The term "ulcerative colitis" is applied to a disease in which a part or whole of the mucosa of the large bowel becomes diffusely inflamed with a haemorrhagic type of inflammation, which may progress to ulceration.'[1]

The symptoms of the disease include diarrhoea and the passage of blood and mucus through the rectum. There may be complications of the disease and the patient may become very ill due to anaemia, hypoproteinaemia and disturbance in the body's fluid and electrolyte balance. During a severe attack the patient may pass 20 or more stools each day resulting in acute illness and very poor quality of life.

Medical treatment of ulcerative colitis usually includes sulpha-salazine (Salazopyrin) and corticosteroids (prednisolone) administered either systemically or locally per rectum. However, about

20–25% of patients need to be treated with surgery.[1] The degree of colonic involvement appears to affect the requirement for surgery, from 2% in patients with proctitis to 33% in extensive disease.[2] Surgery usually involves the removal of the whole colon and creation of an ileostomy. However, more recently there have been surgical developments which avoid the patient having a permanent stoma. (See Chapter 3.)

The aetiology of ulcerative colitis is still unknown. Various factors have been considered including infection, diet, psychological influences and immunological factors.[3] The disease can develop at any age but it most commonly develops in young adults, the most frequently affected age group being 20–39 years.[4] Slightly more women than men are affected in a ratio of 4:3, except in childhood where the sex ratio is reversed.[5]

The disease usually takes the form of acute exacerbations interspersed with periods of remission. However, there are various situations when surgery to cure the disease is indicated.

Elective surgery

Failure of medical treatment. Severe disease with frequent acute attacks which are not controlled by medical treatment, resulting in a poor quality of life for the patient.

Risk of colonic malignancy. It is recognized that patients with ulcerative colitis have an increased risk of developing colonic carcinoma[3] but the reports on this risk appear to vary from 1.7%[7] to 11.1%[6] possibly due to the different types of case studied. Factors that appear to influence the development of carcinoma are:

1. *The duration of the colitis:* It is generally found that the incidence of carcinoma increases with the duration of symptoms of colitis. One study calculated that the risk of developing cancer is 20 times as high in those who have colitis for 20 years or more as it is for those who have had colitis for under five years.[8]
2. *The age of the patient at onset of colitis:* The risk of developing carcinoma is much increased in patients whose ulcerative colitis developed in childhood. The incidence

appears to decrease proportionately with the age of the patient at the onset of colitis, the risk being minimal in those developing colitis over the age of 60 years.[8]

3. *The extent of colonic involvement:* Studies have shown that colitis which is confined to the rectum and left side of the colon rarely predisposes to malignancy; the danger appears to exist mainly in patients with total colonic involvement.[7]

Many surgeons used to recommend proctocolectomy with ileostomy to patients with ulcerative colitis that had affected the whole of the colon for 10 years or more.[3] However, more recent studies have now revealed that it is possible to predict the malignant potential of long-standing extensive colitis by assessing the degree of dysplasia in the colonic mucosal biopsies.[9] In view of this evidence many surgeons have now adopted a more conservative approach of management provided the patient has multiple colonoscopic and rectal biopsies performed annually.

Retardation of growth and development. In children and adolescents with severe ulcerative colitis physical retardation may occur. The prognosis is often poor in children with colitis and surgery is often indicated.[10]

Extra-colonic manifestations of the disease. Colitic arthritis, ankylosing spondylitis and sacroileitis are all recognized in association with ulcerative colitis and are usually seen to regress following curative surgery. Skin lesions such as erythema nodosum and pyoderma gangrenosum are also well-recognized complications of the disease, as are eye complications such as iritis. These conditions usually indicate active disease process in the colon; some may regress but the severity of the symptoms may be influential when curative surgery is being considered.

Emergency surgery

Failure to achieve remission of an acute attack. If medical management fails to achieve a remission in a severe attack of ulcerative colitis then surgery may be recommended. There is a greater likelihood of having to resort to urgent operation if:

- There is total bowel involvement.
- There is rapid onset of a very severe attack.
- The patient is aged less than 20 years.
- The patient is aged over 60 years.[3]

Sudden deterioration in patient's condition. Emergency surgery may be indicated at any stage of the disease in response to a sudden deterioration in the patient's general condition[3]—which may result from one of the complications below.

Perforation of the colon. Any severe attack of ulcerative colitis may lead to perforation of the colon with severe peritonitis. In these cases the only hope of saving the patient is to perform an emergency colectomy.[1]

Toxic megacolon. In a severe attack of ulcerative colitis the colon may dilate greatly and the patient's general condition deteriorate. This situation can rapidly lead to colonic perforation. Regular girth measurement and daily abdominal X-rays to assess whether there is any increase in colonic proportions is advisable in an acute attack of ulcerative colitis if toxic megacolon is suspected.

Severe haemorrhage. Severe uncontrollable haemorrhage from the bowel may occur which cannot be readily replaced by blood transfusion and thus endangers the patient's life.

In these situations rapid surgical intervention is indicated. Joint management and consultation between physicians and surgeons facilitates appropriate decision making.

Crohn's disease

Crohn's disease is a chronic, progressive, granulomatous, inflammatory disorder which may affect any part of the alimentary tract from mouth to anus.[11] Dr B.B. Crohn first described the disease in 1932 as occurring only in the terminal ileum.[12] However, it is now accepted that this was incorrect.

The symptoms of the disease are similar to those seen in ulcerative colitis, including diarrhoea, anaemia and weight loss. Abdominal pain is more pronounced in Crohn's disease than ulcerative colitis as are anal lesions, e.g. fissures, abscesses and fistulae. Fistula formation, either internal or external, is a feature of the disease possibly caused by leakage via a deep fissure in the bowel wall forming an inflammatory mass in which abscesses develop. These abscesses may burst into an adjacent organ or the exterior of the body. Nutritional support in this situation is of paramount importance. Crohn's disease can affect any part of the alimentary tract and it is characterized by areas of healthy intestine being interspersed with areas of disease which are known as 'skip lesions'. The quality of life for patients with Crohn's disease can be very poor, due to general ill health, pain, diarrhoea, malnutrition and imbalance in the body's fluids and electrolytes.

The medical treatment for Crohn's disease includes sulphasalazine (Salazopyrin), corticosteroids (prednisolone) and immunosuppressives (azathioprine); the patient may also require nutritional support. The incidence of Crohn's disease particularly in the large bowel appears to be increasing[13,14] but the underlying cause of the condition is still unknown. Various factors have been considered in association with aetiology, which include genetic, immunological, environmental, dietary and microbiological influences. The disease can occur at any age but onset is most common between 20 and 40 years.

Surgical intervention in Crohn's disease may be indicated to resect severely affected areas and deal with acute complications. The exact nature of the surgery undertaken in Crohn's disease is dependent upon the site and extent of the lesions. The patient may have an ileostomy or, in some cases, a colostomy if the severe disease is localized to the rectum. Surgery will rarely bring about a cure as recurrence after operation is common, being reported at up to 50% after 10 years usually at a site just proximal to the anastomosis.[11] Further lesions can also develop elsewhere in the digestive tract.

The indications for surgery in Crohn's disease are as follows:

Elective surgery

Deteriorating general health: The severity of symptoms and the patient's general condition are usually assessed by the surgeon.

Chronic ill health or the development of complications not responsive to conservative treatment may influence the decision to operate. This is weighed against the possible improvement after operation and the risk of recurrence. It is, however, reported that as many as 93% of patients suffering from Crohn's disease of the small intestine eventually require surgical intervention.[15] Those with the disease of the large bowel appear to require surgery less frequently.[14]

Retardation of growth and development: In cases of Crohn's disease in children approaching puberty, elective resection of major lesions is often undertaken more quickly due to the risk of retardation in physical development if the disease remains.[14]

Fistula formation. Fistulae may occur:

1. Between adjacent loops of bowel.
2. Between the bowel and the bladder.
3. Between the bowel and the vagina.
4. Between the bowel and the body's exterior.

The occurrence of fistulae may necessitate surgical intervention.

Intestinal obstruction. In Crohn's disease intestinal obstruction due to stricture formation is usually subacute. Total occlusion of the bowel is rare and the obstruction is usually managed conservatively allowing for elective surgery if appropriate.[11]

Abscess formation. Abscesses develop in 15–25% of cases from deep ulcers that have penetrated the bowel wall.[16] These abscesses may extend widely and predispose to fistulae.

Severe anal disease. Severe Crohn's disease of the rectum and anus involving abscess formation and fistulae may necessitate excision of the diseased area.

Colonic malignancy. There is an increased risk of colonic malignancy developing in Crohn's disease. Surgery would, however, usually only be undertaken in cases where biopsies showed severe dysplasia.

Emergency surgery

Perforation. Perforation is most commonly seen in the terminal ileum, just proximal to a stricture. If this occurs peritonitis will develop. It is usual to exteriorize the bowel proximal to the perforation as primary anastomosis is not often recommended.[11] A perforation can reseal leaving a 'walled-off' abscess or an area of inflammation.

Toxic megacolon. Severe acute attacks of Crohn's disease may progress to a fulminating, disintegrative stage, terminating in dilatation. This can predispose to perforation.

Severe haemorrhage. If severe haemorrhage occurs the most common site is the terminal ileum. If the blood loss cannot be readily replaced with transfusion then surgery is indicated.

Familial polyposis

Familial intestinal polyposis is a hereditary disease characterized by the development within the colon of large numbers of adenomatous polyps.[17] They are known to be premalignant and if left untreated cancer of the colon will almost certainly develop.[18] The condition is inherited as an autosomal dominant gene, so that 50% of offspring will receive the gene.[19] Familial polyposis is said to be one of the most clearly defined precancerous diseases known in medicine.[17] Patients with a family history of the disease should be examined regularly by sigmoidoscopy to elicit the presence of polyps. The disease commonly develops in the teens and early twenties and if untreated malignancy will occur by the age of about 35 years. If polyps are detected then total colectomy is essential but ileostomy may be avoided. (See Chapter 3.)

In some patients suffering from the disease there may be associated multiple sebaceous or epidermoid cysts, bony exostoses or fibrous connective tissue tumours. This condition is known as Gardner's syndrome and occurs in about 16.4% of patients with familial polyposis.[20]

Carcinoma of the colon

Carcinoma is a malignant disorder of cell growth arising in epitheal disease. Colorectal cancer is the second most common cause of death from malignancy in Britain, Australia and New Zealand, and in the United States it has become the most common.[21] There has been little change in the figures for the number of deaths from this disease in the last 40 years.[22] The incidence throughout the world varies considerably but it is more prevalent in Westernized countries.[23]

The site incidence studies show that the rectum is by far the most common site for carcinoma to occur.[24,25] The tumour site distribution of a survey of 1939 patients is shown in Fig. 7.[25]

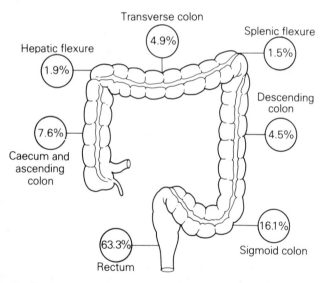

Fig. 7. *Site incidence of large bowel carcinoma (from McDermott et al.[25]).*

Carcinoma of the colon is predominantly a disease of later life, the majority of patients being between 50 and 70 years. The aetiology of the disease is not fully understood but there appear to be strong links with environmental factors and diet.[26] Familial polyposis coli is also known to predispose to colonic cancer.[18]

The type of carcinoma, the degree of differentiation and the grading, as described below, have a direct implication upon the prognosis. There may be one of four macroscopic appearances:

1. *Ulcerating*—the growth presents as a malignant ulcer with raised irregular edges and a sloughing base.
2. *Polypoid*—the growth produces a large fungating mass which protrudes into the bowel lumen.
3. *Annular*—the growth extends around the bowel wall and may result in stenosis.
4. *Diffusely infiltrating*—the growth produces a diffuse thickening of the intestinal wall.

Microscopically the cancer can be described in three classifications:

1. *Well differentiated*—closely resembling parent tissue.
2. *Moderately differentiated*—losing the feature of the parent tissue.
3. *Poorly differentiated*—having no resemblance to parent tissue, being completely anaplastic.

In Britain colonic carcinomas are commonly graded in four categories: *Grade A*—confined to bowel wall; *Grade B*—extending beyond the bowel wall; *Grade C*—involvement of lymph nodes; *Grade D*—distant metastasis, e.g. in the liver.

Colonic carcinoma can spread in five ways:

- Through the bowel wall, i.e. direct spread to surrounding structures.
- Through the peritoneal cavity.
- By way of the lymphatics.
- By means of the bloodstream.
- By implantation to a raw surface or suture line in the bowel.[22]

The symptoms of carcinoma of the rectum or colon may include:

- Alteration in bowel habit, i.e. constipation, diarrhoea or a combination of the two.
- The passage of blood or slime per rectum.
- Abdominal or perineal pain.
- Dyspepsia.
- Flatulent distension.
- Audible bowel sounds.
- Tenesmus.
- Impaired general health, weight loss, decreased strength and anaemia.[27]

Surgery for colonic carcinoma may be curative or palliative. In curative surgery the whole tumour is removed together with an adequate margin of healthy bowel and the corresponding lymphatics. This procedure may involve a temporary or permanent colostomy depending upon the site of the growth and the specific procedure. Palliative surgery may be undertaken if a complete excision of the growth is not possible, to relieve symptoms, prevent obstruction and improve the patient's quality of life. Palliative procedures frequently include the formation of a stoma.

Diverticular disease

Diverticular disease is a condition in which small pouches (diverticulae) are seen protruding from the bowel wall. It is recognized that patients with such disease have an increased intraluminal pressure[28] which causes herniation of the colonic mucosa through the weak spots in the bowel wall where blood vessels enter. For this reason diverticulae are constantly seen distributed in rows between the taenia coli.[29] These pouches may become inflamed in which case the term 'diverticulitis' is applied to the condition.

Studies show that the condition rarely affects patients under 30 years of age, the most commonly affected age group being those between 60 and 90 years.[30] As many as 50% of patients aged 80–90 years have been shown to have this disease.[31] The disease most commonly affects the sigmoid colon but in some 16% of cases the whole colon may be affected.[32] Diverticular disease is thought to result from the excessive effect of segmentation which is normally a mechanism to halt the faecal stream or move it distally or proximally.[28] Lack of dietary fibre increases faecal transit time allowing more water absorption and thus resulting in the formation of smaller firmer stools which require more contraction to expel and stimulates excessive segmentation. This, in turn, produces high pressure and induces the formation of diverticulae.[33] The ingestion of bran has shown to reduce intestinal transit time.[34] Epidemiological evidence has been produced suggesting that lack of bulk (particularly high fibre cereal) is the most important factor producing diverticular disease in the Western community.

Many patients with diverticular disease are unaware of its existence and suffer few symptoms. Others complain of chronic or intermittent symptoms which include abdominal pain or discomfort, distension and alteration of bowel habit, usually constipation.[36]

The disease is usually treated by advising the patient to take a diet high in fibre with additional bran. Some doctors also prescribe bulk laxatives such as sterculia (Normacol) or ispaghula husk (Isogel) and many patients find this management satisfactory. Antispasmodics such as mebeverine hydrochloride (Colofac) may also be prescribed prior to recommending surgical treatment.

Indications for surgery

Repeated acute attacks of diverticulitis. Patients who suffer repeated acute attacks of diverticulitis are often best treated by elective surgery before severe complications occur.[29]

Colonic obstruction. Chronic inflammation may result in stricture formation which causes intestinal obstruction and usually merits surgery. The condition may be acute or chronic. Acute cases may require staged operation.

Fistula formation. Colocutaneous or colovesical festulae are usually considered to be indications for staged surgical intervention, provided the patient is generally fit. A colovesical fistula is very dangerous due to the risk of ascending urinary tract infection.

Abscess formation. An abscess may form in and around the diverticulum as a result of infection, and may predispose to purulent peritonitis.

Perforation of diverticulum. Faecal peritonitis may result from the perforation of a diverticulum allowing the spillage of faeces from the colon into the peritoneal cavity.

Severe chronic symptoms. Patients with chronic symptoms of diverticular disease despite taking a high fibre diet and medication usually enjoy good results following surgical resection, provided they are not also suffering from irritable bowel syndrome.

In cases where surgery is undertaken electively and the patient is adequately prepared, resection of the affected portion of bowel is usually the procedure of choice. In some cases a defunctioning colostomy to protect the anastomosis is indicated. (See Chapter 3.) In emergency cases or in the presence of a fistula a defunctioning stoma is commonly fashioned until definitive surgery can be undertaken. In most cases the stoma is temporary.

Colonic obstruction

Two common causes of colonic obstruction are carcinoma, which has already been discussed, and volvulus. Severe faecal impaction may also result in obstruction.

Volvulus

A sigmoid volvulus occurs when the gut becomes twisted on its mesenteric axis resulting in obstruction. In the UK about 4% of patients presenting with intestinal obstruction are suffering from sigmoid volvulus.[37] However, the condition is more common in other countries, such as Russia and India.[38] The condition commonly affects the older age group, particularly those with associated medical and psychiatric disorders, and these patients have commonly come from long-term care institutions.[37]

It is often possible to decompress and untwist the bowel by passing a rubber tube via a sigmoidoscope. Elective surgery is then usually undertaken at a later date to prevent recurrence. However, if this tube does not achieve decompression or gangrene is suspected then surgery is indicated. This usually involves a two-stage procedure such as Hartmann's operation or a Bloch–Paul–Mikulicz procedure.

Severe faecal impaction

Severe faecal impaction can cause intestinal obstruction and occasionally surgery involving a stoma is necessary, particularly in conditions where the colon above the impaction is grossly distended. In this situation perforation of the colon can sometimes occur.

Bowel ischaemia

If the blood supply to the gastrointestinal tract is compromised necrosis begins at the innermost layer of the mucosa and spreads outwards; gangrene will ensue within 5–6 hours. The severity and extent of ischaemic damage is dependent upon the size of the blocked vessel and the duration of the blockage. The area of gut affected is dependent upon the specific vessel involved. Other factors such as haemoglobin level, the presence of heart disease, the pattern of the individual's collateral blood supply and the gut's bacterial population are influential in the outcome of ischaemic damage.

Bowel ischaemia can result from a variety of causes, such as:

- Surgical trauma.
- Embolus.
- Diseases that produce inflammation of minor arteries resulting in mucosal damage, e.g. systemic lupus erythematosus or rheumatoid arthritis.
- Impairment in circulation resulting from cardiovascular disease.
- Intestinal obstruction.

Bowel ischaemia may be considered in two categories: massive necrosis and ischaemic colitis.

Massive necrosis (gangrene)

This usually occurs in the older age groups and patients frequently suffer from cardiovascular disease. The patient is generally extremely ill and requires resuscitation prior to laparotomy. Surgery commonly involves excising the necrotic segment of bowel. Anastomosis is not usually attempted; the proximal end of bowel being exteriorized as a stoma. If it has been necessary to excise a large portion of small bowel then nutritional and metabolic problems can occur.

Ischaemic colitis (non-gangrenous)

This is a milder form of ischaemia and the patient usually has left-sided peritonitis, diarrhoea and rectal bleeding. Many cases settle with conservative treatment and it is rare for gangrene to occur. Some patients develop a fibrous stricture which may require surgical resection only if it gives rise to symptoms that cause distress.

Anorectal incontinence

Continence is dependent upon a balance between faecal consistency and the efficiency of anal sphincter mechanisms. Fluid stools resulting from a disorder of the large bowel such as inflammatory bowel disease or gastroenteritis may not be contained by the anal sphincter resulting in incontinence. Disruption of the anal sphincters may result from:

1. Trauma, e.g. impalement injury or obstetric accident.
2. Impaired efficiency, e.g. in cases of rectal prolapse or anal neoplasm preventing the anal canal flattening.
3. Muscular disorders, e.g. impairment of smooth and striated muscle function.
4. Congenital anorectal anomalies.

Many of these conditions are treated by surgical sphincter repair but if this is unsuccessful the patient may enjoy a much improved quality of life following the fashioning of a proximal diverting colostomy. The treatment of established anorectal incontinence depends upon the cause and severity of the disorder.[39]

Trauma

Trauma or injury to the abdomen may result in perforation of the intestine. This condition may be seen following road traffic accidents, industrial injury, stabbing or bullet wounds. Surgery is usually undertaken to defunction the bowel since leakage of faeces must be stopped as a priority. A temporary stoma proximal to the injury is usually created prior to closing the perforation. If the injury involves the small intestine then resection and primary anastomosis may be performed.

Irradiation damage

The bowel is recognized as being sensitive to irradiation. Most cases of rectal damage due to irradiation are associated with the treatment of gynaecological or bladder cancer. The symptoms of such damage are usually diarrhoea and abdominal cramps in the early stages, but later complications can occur such as stricture, ulceration with fistulae formation haemorrhage or necrosis.

Patients' tolerance to radiation varies but one author reports that: 'With present techniques patients who are given more than 6000 rads on the bowel run a considerable risk of developing severe complications.'[40] These complications frequently result in the patient requiring a stoma.

CONDITIONS THAT MAY REQUIRE URINARY DIVERSION

Some of the conditions that require urinary diversion are discussed later in this chapter since they are paediatric conditions, such as: bladder exstrophy; cloacal exstrophy; fistulae; and neurogenic bladder as a result of spina bifida. Other conditions that may predispose to urinary diversion are as follows:

Bladder cancer

In England and Wales bladder cancer accounts for about 7% of all male cancers and 2.5% of all female cancers. It rarely occurs under the age of 50 years, but after this age there is a sharp rise in incidence.[41] The most likely initiators of bladder cancer are diverse; they are environmental factors to which we are exposed as a result of our diet, social habits, or working conditions.[42] Some examples are industrial chemicals,[43,44] cigarette smoking particularly in men,[45] coffee drinking,[46] and excessive use of artificial sweeteners.[47]

Bladder cancers are categorized into 'T' categories of the TNM classifications (Tumour, Node, Metastasis) described in 1978 by Union Internationale Contre Cancer (UICC) as follows (Fig. 8):

TIS   Flat carcinoma, the mucosa appears abnormal.
Ta   Superficial carcinoma.
T_1 Superficial carcinoma with invasive potential.
T_2 Invasive into superficial muscle.
T_3 Invasive into deep muscle.
T_4 Invasive into other organs.

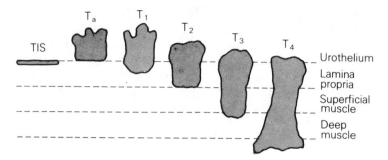

Fig. 8. *'T' categories of bladder cancer.*

The treatment of bladder cancer is usually dependent upon the category of the tumour. However, involvement of lymph nodes and metastasis are also influential. Some superficial tumours are manageable by diathermy, transurethral resection or chemotherapy. T_2 tumours require deep transurethral resection. These superficial tumours require monitoring regularly on a three-monthly basis. If conservative treatment fails then radiotherapy or cystectomy may be indicated. Radical cystectomy is usually undertaken for T_3 tumours often coupled with radiotherapy and cytotoxic drugs. Studies have shown that if the patient is given preoperative radiotherapy the survival rate is improved.[48] In the case of T_4 tumours treatment is usually palliative; this may include radiotherapy if the patient's general condition is satisfactory. Few patients with T_4 tumours survive for longer than one year.[49]

Following cystectomy it is necessary to divert the urine most commonly via an intestinal conduit. (See Chapter 3.)

Contracted bladder

Patients with interstitial cystitis or healed bladder tuberculosis experience intense pain and intolerable frequency of micturition as the bladder becomes fibrosed. Urinary diversion may be undertaken to improve the patient's quality of life.

Incontinence

In some cases where severe incontinence is making the quality of the patient's life intolerable, urinary diversion may be undertaken.

Treatment of urinary incontinence involving less radical intervention such as medication, electronic muscle stimulation or surgical repair is usually attempted. If these fail or are unacceptable to the patient then urinary diversion may be undertaken.

Failure of uretero-colic anastomosis

In cases where uretero-colic anastomosis becomes dangerous due to infection or metabolic complications or the patient is incontinent per rectum, the urinary flow may be diverted by an intestinal conduit.

SUMMARY

Urinary diversion may be indicated if:

1. *The bladder is dangerous*
   (i) Malignancy.
   (ii) Risk of repeated renal infection.
2. *The bladder is useless*
   (i) Neurogenic bladder, e.g. spina bifida.
   (ii) Congenital abnormalities, e.g. exstrophy.
3. *The bladder is a nuisance*
   (i) Severe incontinence.
4. *The bladder is painful*
   (i) Interstitial cystitis.
   (ii) Tuberculosis.
5. *There is failure of uretero-colic anastomosis*
   (i) Becomes dangerous because of infection or metabolic complications.
   (ii) Leads to incontinence per rectum.

PAEDIATRIC CONDITIONS THAT MAY REQUIRE SURGERY INVOLVING A STOMA

Congenital abnormalities

These are malformations that are present in infants from birth.

Anorectal anomalies

Anorectal anomalies are said to occur once in 5000 births. They can be classified into three groups:

1. High anomalies—the abnormality occurs above the pelvic floor.
2. Intermediate anomalies—these abnormalities occur between the other two groups.
3. Low anomalies—the abnormality occurs below the pelvic floor.[50]

Usually only high and intermediate anomalies require surgery involving a stoma. The colostomy is usually temporary to defunction the bowel until the condition is fully assessed and definitive surgery is undertaken.

High anomalies (anorectal agenesis). The bowel ends blindly or by a fistula above the pelvic floor; the anal canal is absent. The rectum usually opens into the prostatic urethra in the male, the posterior fornix of the vagina in the female.

Intermediate anomalies. The group of anomalies which may be described as intermediate are anorectal stenosis, rectobulbar fistula and rectovestibular fistula.

Bladder exstrophy

Bladder exstrophy is a condition in which the anterior wall of the bladder, the roof of the urethra, and parts of the anterior abdominal wall are missing. The pubic bones and the recti abdominales are widely separated.[51] This condition is twice as common in male babies and occurs in different communities between one in 10000 and one in 40000 live births. The size of the exstrophic bladder varies considerably and at birth the exposed mucosa is thin and smooth and the muscular coat is thin and pliable; the organ bulges outwards due to intra-abdominal pressure and can be inverted by digital compression.[52]

In some cases reconstruction of the bladder is possible and continence can be achieved, but this is rare. If it is not possible then urinary diversion is considered. Provided that the upper renal tract is not distended, ureterosigmoidostomy may be the procedure of choice.[53] However, if there is defective anal sphincter control or dilatation in the upper renal tract an external diversion is necessary in the form of an intestinal conduit, or some surgeons prefer an ureterostomy.[52]

Cloacal exstrophy

This is an extreme disorder involving the bladder, ureters, and intestine, all of which are exposed. The condition is often associated with other congenital abnormalities and the baby is often premature, thus not many patients survive. In those that do both a faecal and urinary stoma are required to facilitate elimination.

Other abnormalities of the urinary tract

Urethral-vaginal confluence or cloaca in which there is also recto-vaginal fistula resulting in a single perineal opening leads to urinary incontinence requiring diversion.

Spina bifida

Spina bifida is an abnormality of the central nervous system, which occurs in about 1.5 per 1000 live births. During development a gap

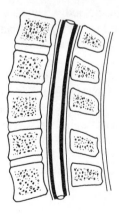

Cross section of
normal spinal column

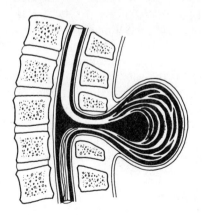

Cross section of
severe spina bifida
(meningomyelocele)

Fig. 9. *Spina bifida.*

occurs in the spinal column through which the contents of the spinal canal may protrude (Fig. 9). There are various degrees of spina bifida and in some cases the nervous control of the bladder is defective (neurogenic bladder). This results in urinary incontinence and stagnation of urine due to incomplete bladder emptying. This predisposes to infections which can eventually involve the kidney and result in renal failure.

In many children with spina bifida bladder expression or intermittent self-catheterization is taught with very successful results. However, in some it is eventually necessary to divert the urine to the exterior, usually via an intestinal conduit.

Hirschsprung's disease

Hirschsprung's disease is a congenital defect of the large intestine, where the network of nerves in a segment of the intestine is incomplete and, therefore, the muscles do not work. The contents of the intestine are held up at this point and the intestine becomes very distended. The disease occurs in one per 5000 live births and the ratio of male to female is 5:1. The aetiology is not known but a genetic factor has been suggested. The disease is a congenital, functional intestinal obstruction in which the normally innervated bowel proximal to the aganglionic segment becomes grossly dilated (megacolon). The disease is often suspected when faecal elimination is impaired. Abdominal distension is often present and peristalsis may be visible. Feeding may be difficult to establish and bile-stained vomiting may occur after feeds.

In the neonatal period a colostomy is usually performed immediately proximal to the aganglionic segment to relieve the obstruction. In some cases of high segment Hirschsprung's disease an ileostomy may be fashioned. At a later date definitive surgery involving a 'pull-through' technique is often undertaken and the colostomy subsequently closed.

Other paediatric conditions

Necrotizing enterocolitis

This condition most commonly occurs in premature babies, more of whom have been surviving in recent years due to improved clinical expertise and technology.

The gut becomes necrotic and bacterial infections occur. The extent of the mucosal lesions varies from a few centimetres to the whole gut from duodenum to rectum. The lesions may extend through the muscle wall resulting in perforation.[54]

Treatment involves discontinuing oral feeding and maintaining fluid and nutritional requirements parenterally; antibiotic therapy is given and the conditions closely monitored. Surgery may be required if the bowel perforates or where there is persistent obstruction or strictures. This often involves exteriorizing the gut at either side of the non-viable segment. Surgery to close enterostomies is usually performed after recovery.

Meconium ileus

Cystic fibrosis is a multi-organ disease probably due to a primary disorder of the exocrine and mucus secreting glands, resulting in the production of very thick mucus which may block ducts.[55] Diagnosis of the disease is made by sampling the sweat from the child. The disease affects the pancreas which produces enzymes that travel to the duodenum via small ducts. The ducts are protected from digestion by mucous secretions. In cystic fibrosis the mucus is very thick and sticky and may block the duct. Digestive enzymes are then unable to escape with resultant self-digestion and cyst formation. The cyst fluid is subsequently absorbed by the body resulting in fibrosis. This can result in substantial injury to the pancreas, thus there will not be enough pancreatic enzyme to digest the meconium.

This condition results in the meconium being very thick and tenacious and may result in intestinal obstruction, perforation and peritonitis. Surgery may be required involving an end-to-side (Bishop-Koop) anastomosis to relieve the obstruction and an ileostomy is fashioned. In cases of perforation emergency surgery is necessary. The child will be treated by giving pancreatic enzymes orally with feeds and the ileostomy will, subsequently, be closed.

Trauma

Trauma or injury resulting in damage to gastrointestinal tract may require surgery involving a stoma. Intestinal injury may result from severe non-accidental injury.

REFERENCES

1. Truelove, S.C. (1984) *Ulcerative Colitis*. Update Postgraduate Publication. 4
2. Ritchie, J.K., Powell-Tuck, J. & Lennard-Jones, J.E. (1978) Clinical outcome of the first ten years of ulcerative colitis and proctitis. *Lancet ii*, 1140.
3. Goligher, J.C. (1984) *Surgery of the Anus, Rectum and Colon*, 5th edn. Chap. 22, pp. 805–970. London: Baillière Tindall.
4. Watts, J., et al. (1966) The long-term prognosis of ulcerative colitis. *British Medical Journal, 1*, 1447.
5. Canby, J.P. & Mehchop, F.H. (1964) Ulcerative colitis in children. *American Journal of Gastro-enterology, 42*, 66.
6. De Dombal, F.T., Watts, J.M., Watkinson, G. & Goligher, J.C. (1966) Local complications of ulcerative colitis: stricture, pseudopolyposis and carcinoma of the colon and rectum. *British Medical Journal, i*, 1442.
7. Counsell, P.B., & Dukes, C.E. (1952) The association of chronic ulcerative colitis and carcinoma of the rectum and colon. *British Journal of Surgery, 39*, 485.
8. Edwards, F.C. & Truelove, S.C. (1964) The course and prognosis of ulcerative colitis, part IV; carcinoma of the colon. *Gut, 5*, 1.
9. Lennard-Jones, J.E. et al. (1977) Cancer in colitis—assessment of the individual risks by clinical and histological criteria. *Gastroenterology, 73*, 1280.
10. Welin, S.L. & Grand, R.J. (1977) Severe colitis in children and adolescents: diagnosis course and treatment. *Gastroenterology, 73*, 828.
11. Cunningham, I.G.E. (1983) Inflammatory Bowel Disease. In *Colorectal Surgery*. Eds. Hughes, E., Cutherbertson, A.M., & Killingbeck, M.K. Chap. 24, p. 265. Churchill Livingstone.
12. Crohn, B.B., Ginzburg, L. & Oppenheimer, G.P. (1932) Regional ileitis, pathological and clinical entity. *Journal of the American Medical Association, 99*, 1323–1329.
13. Devlin, H.B., Datta, D., & Dellipiani, A.W. (1980) The incidence and prevalence of inflammatory bowel disease in North Tees Health District. *World Journal of Surgery, 4*, 183–193.
14. Goligher, J.C. (1984) *Surgery of the Anus, Rectum and Colon*, 5th edn. Chap. 23, pp. 971–1017. London: Baillière Tindall.
15. Truelove, S.C. & Pena, A.S. (1976) Course and prognosis of Crohn's disease. *Gut, 17*, 192.
16. Steinberg, D.M., Cooke, W.T., & Alexander-Williams, J. (1973) Abscess and fistula in Crohn's disease. *Gut, 14*, 865–869.
17. Goligher, J.C. (1984) *Surgery of the Anus, Rectum and Colon*, 5th edn. Chap. 15, pp. 358–425 London: Baillière Tindall.
18. Bussey, H.J.R. (1975) *Familial Polyposis Coli*. Johns Hopkins University Press.
19. Pihl, E.A.V., & Penfold, J.C.B. (1983) Benign tumours of the colon and rectum. In *Colorectal Surgery*. Eds. Hughes, E., Cuthbertson, A.M., & Killingbeck, M.C. Chap 30, pp 326–336. Churchill Livingstone.
20. Lockhart-Mummery, H.E. (1967) Intestinal Polyposis: the present position. *Proceedings of the Royal Society of Medicine, 60*, 381.
21. McDermott, F.C. (1983) Colorectal carcinoma, general features and pathology. In *Colorectal Surgery*. Eds. Hughes, E., Cutherbertson, A.M. & Killingbeck, M.K. Chap. 31, pp 336–346. Churchill Livingstone.
22. Goligher, J.C. (1984) *Surgery of the Anus, Rectum and Colon*, 5th edn. Chap 16, pp 426–464. London: Baillière Tindall.

23. Waterhouse, J., Muir, C., Corea, P. & Powell, J. (1976) *Cancer Incidence in Five Continents*, Vol. 3. Lyon. International Agency for Cancer Research.
24. Smiddy, F.G. & Goligher, J.C. (1957) Results of surgery in treatment of cancer of the large intestine. *British Medical Journal, i*, 793.
25. McDermott, F.T., Hughes, E.S.R., Pihl, E., Milne, B.J. & Price, A.B. (1981) Comparative results of surgical management of single carcinoma of the colon and rectum: a series of 1930 patients managed by one surgeon. *British Journal of Surgery, 68*, 850–855.
26. Burkitt, D. (1975) *Benign and Malignant Tumours of the Large Bowel. Refined Carbohydrate Foods and Disease: Some Implications of Dietary Fibre.* Eds. Burkitt, D., & Trowell, H.C., Chap. 10, pp 117–134. London: Academic Press.
27. Goligher, J.C. (1984) *Surgery of the Anus, Rectum and Colon*, 5th edn. Chap. 17, pp 465–484. London: Baillière Tindall.
28. Painter, N.S. & Truelove, S.C. (1964) The intraluminal pressure patterns in diverticulosis of the colon. *Gut, 5*, 201–213.
29. Hughes, E., Cuthbertson, A.M., & Killingbeck, M.K. (1983) Diverticular disease of the colon. In *Colorectal Surgery*. Chap. 25, pp 289–308. Churchill Livingstone.
30. Parks, T.G. (1969) Natural history of diverticular disease of the colon. A review of 521 cases. *British Medical Journal, iv*, 639–642.
31. Parks, T.G. (1968) Post mortem studies on the colon with special reference to diverticular disease. *Proceedings of the Royal Society of Medicine. 61*, 932.
32. Hughes, L.E. (1969) Post mortem of diverticular disease of the colon. *Gut, 10*, 336–351.
33. Painter, N.S., Truelove, S.C., Ardran, G.M., & Tuckey, M. (1965) Segmentation and the localisation of intraluminal pressures in the human colon, with specific reference to the pathogenesis of the colonic diverticula. *Gastroenterology, 49*, 169–177.
34. Findlay, J.M., Smith, A.N., Mitchell, W.D., Anderson, A.J.B., & Eastwood, M.A. (1974) Effects of unprocessed bran on colon function in normal subjects and in diverticular disease. *Lancet, i*, 146–9.
35. Painter, N.S., & Burkitt, D.P. (1975) Diverticular disease of the colon, a 20th century problem. *Clinics in Gastroenterology, 4*, 3–21.
36. Goligher, J.C. (1984) Diverticulosis and diverticulitis of the colon. In *Surgery of the Anus, Rectum and Colon*, 5th edn. Chap. 29, pp 1083–1116. London: Baillière Tindall.
37. Anderson, J.R. & Lee, D. (1981) The management of acute sigmoid volvulus. *British Journal of Surgery, 68*, 117.
38. Sinha, R.S. (1969) A clinical appraisal of volvulus of the pelvic colon with special reference to aetiology and treatment. *British Journal of Surgery, 56*, 838.
39. Polglase, A.L. (1983) Anorectal incontinence. In *Colorectal Surgery*. Eds. Hughes, E., Cuthbertson, A.M. & Killingbeck, M.K. Chap. 21, pp 215–219. Churchill Livingstone.
40. Hughes, E., Cuthbertson, A.M. & Killingbeck, M.K. (1983) Irradiation damage of the bowel. In *Colorectal Surgery*. Eds. Hughes, E., Cuthbertson, A.M. & Killingbeck, M.K. Chap. 26, 309–312. Churchill Livingstone.
41. Pugh, R.C.B. (1982) Histopathology. In *Urology*, 2nd edn. Ed. Chisholm, G.D., & Williams, D.I. Chap. 84, pp 701–711. Heinemann.
42. Hicks, R.M. (1982) The development of bladder cancer. *Urology*, 2nd edn. Eds. Chisholm, G.D., & Williams, D.I. Chap. 85, pp 711–722. Heinemann.

43. Davies, J.M. (1965) Bladder tumours in the electric cables industry. *Lancet, ii*, 143.
44. Doll, R., et al. (1965) Mortality of gas workers, with special reference to cancers of the lung and bladder. Chronic bronchitis and pneumoconiosis. *British Journal of Industrial Medicine, 22*, 1.
45. Tyrrell, A.B., McCaughey, W.T.E. & MacAirt, J.G. (1971) Occupational and non-occupational factors associated with vesical neoplasm in Ireland. *Journal of the Irish Medical Association, 64*, 213.
46. Howe, G.R. et al. (1980) Tobacco use, occupation, coffee, various nutrients and bladder cancer. *Journal of the National Cancer Institution, 64*, 701.
47. Hoover, R. (1980) Saccharin-bitter aftertaste. *New England Journal of Medicine, 302*, 573.
48. Whitmore, W.F. (1980) Integrated irradiation and cystectomy for bladder cancer. *British Journal of Urology, 52*,
49. Riddle, P.R. (1980) Surgery of bladder cancer. In *Urology*. Ed. Chisholm, G.D. Chap. 13, pp 192–205. Heinemann.
50. Nixon, H. (1984) Congenital deformities of the anorectal region. In *Surgery of the Anus, Rectum and Colon*. Ed. Goligher, J.C. Chap. 11, pp 285–304. London: Baillière Tindall.
51. Badenoch, A.W. (1974) Congenital anomalies. In *Manual of Urology*. 2nd edn. Chap. 5, pp 97–143. Heinemann.
52. Johnston, J.H. (1982) The exstrophic anomalies. In *Paediatric Urology*, 2nd edn. Ed. Innes Williams, D., & Johnston, J.H. Chap. 25, p 300. London: Butterworth Scientific.
53. Rickwood, A.M.K. (1982) Urinary diversion in children. In *Urinary Diversion*. Ed. Hendley Ashken, M. Chap. 2, p 36. Springer Verlag.
54. Dickson, J.A.S. (1977) Surgical emergencies in the first few weeks of life. *Essentials of Paediatric Gastroenterology*. Ed. Harries, J.T. Chap. 4, pp 63–88. Churchill Livingstone.
55. McCollum, J.P.K. & Harries, J.T. (1977) Disorders of the pancreas. In *Essentials of Paediatric Gastroenterology*. Ed. Harries, J.T. Chap. 20, pp 335–354. Churchill Livingstone.

3 Types of stoma and associated surgical procedures

'*Stoma*' is a Greek word meaning mouth or opening. There are three basic types of eliminating stoma:

- Colostomy—an opening into the colon (large bowel).
- Ileostomy—an opening into the ileum (small intestine).
- Urostomy—an opening into the urinary tract.

COLOSTOMY

Colostomies may be permanent or temporary and can be categorized into four types: 'terminal' or 'end' colostomy; loop colostomy; double-barrel colostomy; divided colostomy.

Terminal colostomy

A terminal colostomy is most commonly situated in the left iliac region of the abdomen. The patient can expect to pass a formed motion as water reabsorption is not compromised. The stools have a typically faecal odour. Although the patient has no voluntary control, a terminal colostomy may establish a pattern of defecation, perhaps once or twice daily and pass only flatus at other times. This type of stoma is suitable for management by irrigation. (See Chapter 15.)

The most common surgical procedures which result in the patient having a terminal colostomy are abdominoperineal excision of the rectum and Hartmann's operation.

Abdominoperineal excision of rectum

The most common indication for this procedure is carcinoma of the distal rectum and some carcinomas of the anal canal. The operation was first established in the UK in the early 1900s,[1] but it did not gain popularity until some 20 years later.

In Britain it is usual for two surgeons to work simultaneously via an abdominal and perineal approach with the patient in a Lloyd Davis position; this is known as a synchronous combined excision of rectum. Some surgeons, however, prefer to do both the abdominal and perineal phases. The proximal bowel is brought out onto the abdominal surface as a terminal colostomy (Fig. 10). The perineal incision is either closed with sutures or packed. The excised area of bowel is illustrated in Fig. 10. The availability of automatic stapling devices to facilitate lower anastomosis being safely achieved has decreased the number of patients requiring abdominoperineal excision of rectum.[2,3]

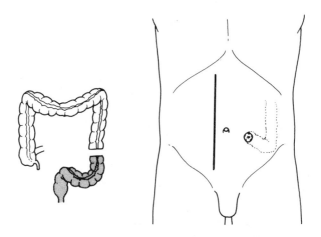

Fig. 10. *Abdominoperineal excision of the rectum.*

Hartmann's operation

Hartmann's operation was originally described in 1923 as a single operation.[4] This involved the upper rectum and sigmoid colon being excised, the rectal stump closed, and a terminal colostomy fashioned as illustrated in Fig. 11. In some cases the procedure may include a second operation to reunite the ends of bowel using a circular stapler.[5] Hartmann's operation may be undertaken for some large bowel cancers (particularly in the emergency

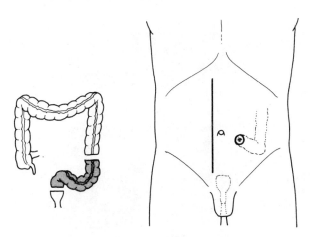

Fig. 11. *Hartmann's operation.*

situation), complicated diverticular disease, or sigmoid volvulus, and results in the patient having a terminal colostomy which may be temporary or permanent.

Loop colostomy

A loop colostomy is most commonly fashioned for the following reasons:

1. To divert the major part of the faecal stream in emergency situations, e.g. distal colonic perforation or trauma.
2. To protect an anastomosis, e.g. following low anterior resection.
3. To decompress the colon in large bowel obstruction.
4. To facilitate healing of colonic disease.

The most common sites for a loop colostomy are the transverse colon to the right of the midline or the sigmoid colon. In this procedure a loop of colon is brought out onto the abdominal surface and supported by a 'rod' or 'bridge'. This may be a glass rod, a piece of rubber tubing, or a specially manufactured plastic support (Fig. 12). The function of this support is to prevent retraction; it usually remains in position for 5–7 days. Once the loop of bowel is supported and the incision closed the colostomy is

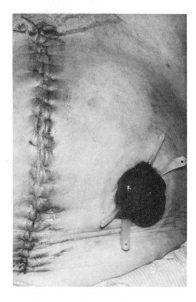

Fig. 12. *A loop colostomy with a plastic support bridge in position.*

opened and the mucosa sutured to the skin's edge. Thus the loop colostomy has two orifices, as shown in Fig. 13: the afferent limb from the digestive tract which is active; and the efferent limb which opens into the 'redundant' colon.

Loop colostomies in the transverse colon tend to be bulky and management problems may occur, particularly while the support bridge is *in situ*. This type of colostomy often acts quite irregularly, passing only a semi-formed motion as some of the colonic water absorption has not taken place. The stools have an offensive faecal odour.

Loop colostomies in the sigmoid colon are a little easier to manage because they occupy a more desirable position and the effluent contains less fluid.

Double-barrelled colostomy (Bloch-Paul-Miculicz)

This type of colostomy may be fashioned in patients with diverticular disease or sigmoid volvulus. The procedure involves resecting the diseased colon and forming a double-barrelled

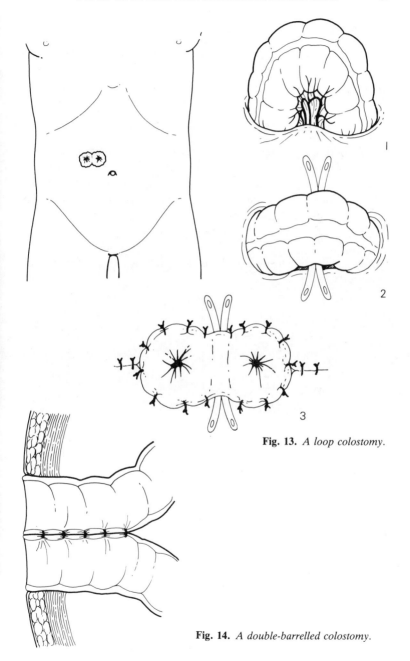

Fig. 13. *A loop colostomy.*

Fig. 14. *A double-barrelled colostomy.*

colostomy by suturing the proximal and distal bowel to form a spur, as illustrated in Fig. 14. The continuity of the bowel can later be restored using a gastrointestinal anastomosis device to 'break the spur'. The colostomy may then close spontaneously or may require a formal closure.

Divided colostomy (Devine operation)

A divided colostomy may be created in cases of obstructing carcinoma or colonic perforation. The procedure involves the excision of the lesion with the proximal bowel being fashioned into a colostomy. The distal end of the colon is fixed to the skin forming a divided colostomy with a bridge of skin between, as shown in Fig. 15. This procedure was first described in 1937 by Devine.[6]

When the colostomy is to be closed, the two ends of bowel are reunited.

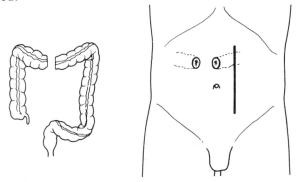

Fig. 15. *A divided colostomy.*

ILEOSTOMY

Ileostomies are frequently permanent but some may be temporary. They can be categorized in two types: terminal ileostomy; and loop ileostomy.

Terminal ileostomy

A terminal ileostomy is constructed when the colon has to be removed, most commonly due to inflammatory bowel disease.

This procedure first became established as a treatment for ulcerative colitis in the 1940s.[7] The first patients with ileostomies encountered serious management problems due to excoriation caused by ileal fluid spilling onto the skin. The technique for fashioning an ileostomy was improved when Brooke described a technique of eversion in 1952[8] (Fig. 16). A terminal ileostomy is

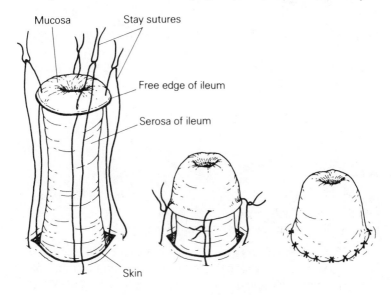

Fig. 16. *A terminal everted ileostomy.*

most commonly situated in the right iliac region of the abdomen. The ileostomy acts frequently, discharging a fluid effluent since there is no colonic fluid reabsorption. Ideally the output should be of 'porridgy' consistency, with the patient passing approximately 350–500 ml per day. The motion does not normally have an offensive odour.[9]

Various surgical procedures may result in the patient having a terminal ileostomy.

Pan-procto colectomy

In this operation the whole colon is excised together with the rectum and anal canal. The terminal ileum is fashioned into an ileostomy which is permanent, as illustrated in Fig. 17.

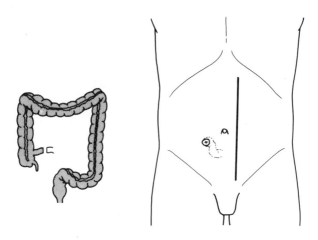

Fig. 17. *Pan-procto colectomy.*

Total colectomy

In this operation the colon is excised but the rectal stump is retained and usually exteriorized as a mucus fistula, as shown in Fig. 18. This operation has several advantages:

1. The anal sphincters are preserved, thus the construction of a pelvic reservoir (pouch) can be considered at a future date.
2. The perineum remains intact, which may be advantageous to female patients of child-bearing age during delivery.

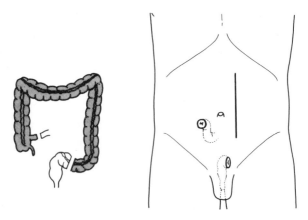

Fig. 18. *Total colectomy; rectal stump retained.*

3. There is no risk of damage to the autonomic nerves supplying the sexual organs, which could result in impotence in the male.
4. The operating time is reduced, which may be critical in an emergency situation when the patient is very ill.

If the rectal stump remains *in situ* for an extended period of time, endoscopic monitoring is essential since this is still a focus of the disease and malignant change may occur.

Loop ileostomy

A loop ileostomy is usually temporary to divert the faecal stream away from:

1. Distal ileorectal or coloanal anastomosis.
2. Anastomoses in an ileal reservoir.
3. Fistulae.
4. Acute Crohn's disease of the rectum or anus.

In cases of inflammatory bowel disease a loop ileostomy should not be constructed on a site that may be subsequently required for a permanent stoma.[9]

A loop ileostomy is constructed in a similar way to a loop colostomy. It is essential that the afferent (active) loop forms a spout to facilitate the collection of effluent without leakage as shown in Fig. 19. Some surgeons now use a subcutaneous

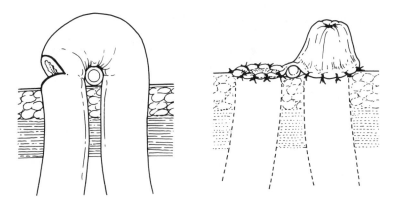

Fig. 19. *A loop ileostomy.*

absorbable oxfibrin support (Biethium by Ethicon) for the loop of intestine in place of a rod.[10] This has the advantage of being below skin level so it does not hamper the application of an appliance.

A loop ileostomy has been shown to be superior to a loop colostomy as a defunctioning stoma because it offers several advantages.[11,12]

- It is a smaller stoma, therefore requires a smaller appliance.
- Loop ileostomy occupies a site which facilitates easier management.
- Effluent has little odour.
- Complications (i.e. prolapse, skin excoriation, minor bleeding, and appliance leakage) occur less often.[11]

UROSTOMY

Diversion of the urinary tract involving a stoma is most commonly permanent. However, some patients who had previously had a urostomy fashioned for a condition that may now be managed by intermittent catheterization may have the procedure reversed (undiversion).[13] There are two common categories of urostomy: intestinal conduit; and ureterostomy.

Intestinal conduit

Ileal conduit

The most popular type of urinary diversion is via an ileal conduit. The operation to divert the urinary flow may also include excision of the bladder (cystectomy), depending upon the predisposing condition. This procedure results in urine from the kidney passing down the ureters into an isolated segment of ileum which acts as a conducting tube (conduit) to the body's surface, as shown in Fig. 20.

To fashion this type of diversion a segment of ileum approximately 10–15 cm long is isolated with its blood supply. Hendry states, 'The ideal length of an ileal conduit is as short as possible to bridge the gap between ureters and anterior abdominal wall, with sufficient to construct a good stoma.'[14] To avoid malabsorption of Vitamin B_{12} and bile salts, the terminal ileum is

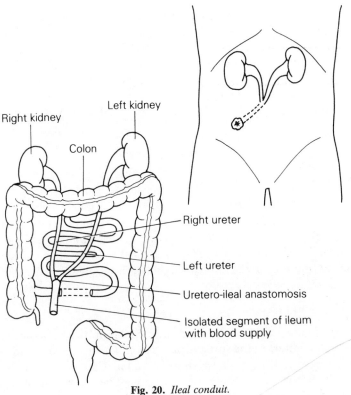

Right kidney

Left kidney

Colon

Right ureter

Left ureter

Uretero-ileal anastomosis

Isolated segment of ileum with blood supply

Fig. 20. *Ileal conduit.*

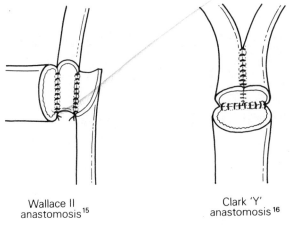

Wallace II
anastomosis[15]

Clark 'Y'
anastomosis[16]

Fig. 21. *Ureters anastomosed to segment of ileum.*

not used. The intestine is then reconstituted by end-to-end anastomosis. The ureters are separated from the bladder and anastomosed to the isolated segment of ileum. Some surgeons implant the ureters separately, others prefer to anastomose the ureters together prior to implantation as described by Wallace[15] or Clarke[16], illustrated in Fig. 21. The conduit is then brought out onto the surface of the abdomen and an everted (Brooke)[8] spout formed.

Colonic conduit

This procedure is very similar to that described to construct an ileal conduit, the difference being that an isolated segment of colon is used to form the conduit. This operation may be used to divert the urinary flow after pelvic exenteration or for some paediatric conditions. The stoma is usually larger than an ileal conduit and sited in the left iliac region of the abdomen.

Ureterostomy

In some cases where there is ureteric dilatation the surgeon may bring the ureters to the surface and form cutaneous ureterostomies as illustrated in Fig. 22. This is more common in paediatric surgery. If only one ureter is dilated the other may be anastomosed to it and a single stoma formed from the dilated ureter.

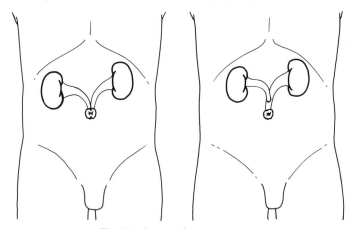

Fig. 22. *Cutaneous ureterostomies.*

ALTERNATIVE PROCEDURES

Circular stapling devices

Prior to the advent of the circular stapling device (gun) considerable difficulties were encountered by surgeons in restoring continuity of the bowel following low anterior resection, especially in the short, obese, male patient with narrow internal pelvic dimensions. This stapling device enables anastomoses to be made quickly and without undue difficulty in less accessible places and is thus ideal for very low colorectal and coloanal anastomoses.[17] However, particular attention is required to the detailed technique in order to obtain good results. Provided that the growth is not so low that excision would impair continence, anterior resection and end-to-end anastomoses using the circular stapling device is now considered as an acceptable sphincter-saving alternative to abdominoperineal excision of rectum of carcinoma.[18]

This procedure involves the lesion being excised after the rectum is mobilized. The device is then inserted through the anus and the anvil (head) is passed up into the proximal colon. A 'purse-string' suture is inserted around each end of the bowel and these are drawn up around the shaft of the gun as shown in Fig. 23. The two ends are then drawn together by closing the device using a winding mechanism. When the 'gun' is fired an anastomosis is made by a double ring of surgical steel staples being automatically inserted. The edges of colon protruding into the instrument's

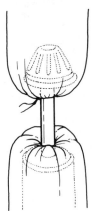

Fig. 23. *Bowel drawn up around the shaft of the 'gun'.*

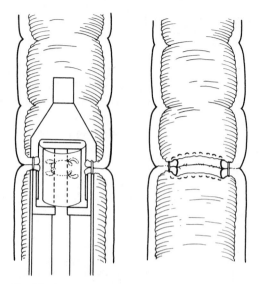

Fig. 24. *Anastomosis made; protruding colon excised.*

lumen and excised by a knife within the device are shown in Fig. 24.

A temporary defunctioning stoma may need to be established to protect the distal anastomosis when:[19]

1. Its integrity is in doubt, i.e. incomplete rings of tissue 'doughnuts' are excised when the instrument is fired.
2. The blood supply is dubious.
3. There is any preoperative contamination.
4. There is a large discrepancy in the diameter of the bowel to be joined.
5. A difficult low anastomosis has been made.

This stapling device is now disposable. It may appear to be expensive but when its cost is equated with the cost of appliances and other services for patients with a permanent colostomy it remains economically viable.[20] Recent research indicates that patients who have undergone excision of low rectal cancer with sphincter-saving resection enjoy a superior quality of life to those who were treated by abdominoperineal excision with permanent colostomy.[21]

Magnetic stoma cap

Another attempt to achieve continence was made using a magnetic plug made of samarium cobalt (Erlangen continent colostomy) to occlude the colostomy. The procedure involves implanting a titanium-coated magnetic ring into the anterior abdominal wall around the colostomy. A corresponding external plastic-coated magnetic cap of opposite polarity is then held in place by the magnetic attraction. The device incorporates a layered charcoal filter-washer which absorbs moisture, filters and releases flatus, and has a cushioning effect on the body surface. (See Fig. 25.) This

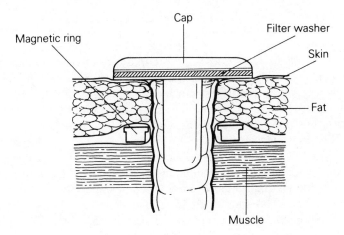

Fig. 25. *Cross-section of colostomy with magnetic sealing device.*

magnetic device has not proved totally effective due to the occurrence of complications such as pressure necrosis between the cap and the ring, infection, faecal seepage, and extrusion of the implanted ring. Some patients complain that the device is heavy and uncomfortable, but others have reported good results.[22]

Other methods of restoring the patient's control over the elimination of faeces and flatus from a terminal colostomy are being researched. Some methods involve occluding the stoma with a tampon or inflatable balloon plug. Other possibilities include attempting to recreate a sphincter around the colostomy.

Ileorectal anastomosis

Ileorectal anastomosis provides an alternative procedure to total proctocolectomy in the treatment of ulcerative colitis. In this procedure the colon is excised and an end-to-end anastomosis is made between the terminal ileum and upper rectum. This operation offers the obvious advantage of conserving the rectum and anal sphincters, so continence is maintained and the patient is spared a permanent ileostomy. However, this procedure is somewhat controversial.[23] There are two main areas of debate: firstly, the quality of life achieved by the patient after surgery; and secondly, the risk of malignancy developing in the retained rectal stump.

Following ileorectal anastomosis all patients pass relatively frequent fluid stools since there is no colonic water reabsorption. Some surgeons claim success in the majority of cases in that the patient opens his bowels not more than six times in 24 hours.[24] However, others report less satisfactory results mainly due to their patients experiencing severe diarrhoea, some requiring a reversal operation and permanent ileostomy.[25]

Research suggests that about 6% of patients will develop rectal carcinoma following ileorectal anastomosis, and this is fatal in the majority of cases.[26] Some surgeons consider this risk too great to justify the procedure unless meticulous postoperative monitoring is arranged. This must include regular sigmoidoscopy at which multiple rectal biopsies are taken to look for signs of severe epithelial dysplasia.[27] The success of the procedure as an alternative surgical treatment for ulcerative colitis is somewhat subjective. Much depends upon the attitude of the patient towards having a stoma. Those individuals who view this prospect with total abhorrence may regard the disadvantages of the procedure as an acceptable price to pay to avoid having a permanent ileostomy.

Kock continent ileostomy

The continent ileostomy which involved an internal reservoir was described by Kock in 1969[27] Following excision of the colon the procedure involves an isoperistaltic pouch being formed from terminal ileum with a capacity of about 500 ml. This provides a reservoir for faeces. The distal outlet of the pouch is closed by a

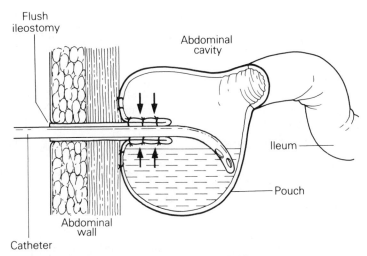

Fig. 26. *A Kock reservoir.*

nipple valve which is fashioned by intussuscepting the bowel into the reservoir as shown in Fig. 26. Pressure within the pouch causes the valve to remain closed; the patient empties the pouch approximately twice daily by passing a semi-rigid catheter through the valve into the reservoir and allowing the faeces to drain.

The advantage of this procedure is that the patient does not have a conventional ileostomy. The outlet of the pouch is usually placed lower on the abdominal wall than a conventional ileostomy, being just above the pubic hairline. The opening is made flush to provide a cosmetically acceptable stoma.[28] However, the nipple valve can be technically difficult to secure and problems can arise if the valve fails to maintain continence due to displacement. Leakage of ileal fluid will then occur and because of the position of the flush stoma secure fitting of an appliance is very difficult.

The procedure is not suitable for patients with Crohn's disease, as recurrence or fistulae may occur within the pouch. This operation may be undertaken at the same time as the colectomy is performed or as a subsequent procedure.

Restorative proctocolectomy with ileal reservoir

This procedure was described by the late Sir Alan Parks in 1978, and for this reason the ileal reservoir is sometimes referred to as

'Parks Pouch'.[29] The operation is only suitable for patients with ulcerative colitis or familial polyposis coli which affects primarily the colonic mucosa. Those with Crohn's disease are excluded due to the risk of fistula formation or recurrence of disease in the reservoir.

The procedure involves excision of the colon between the ileocaecal junction and the lower rectum. A reservoir is then fashioned using a length of terminal ileum which is folded onto itself in a 'J' shape, opened and formed into a pouch (see Fig. 27).

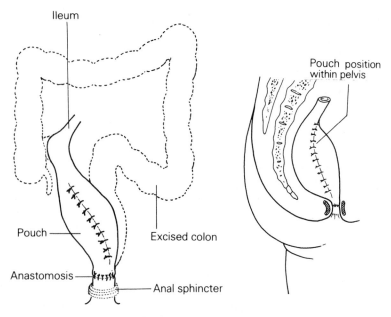

Fig. 27. *An ileal reservoir.*

The mucosa from the rectal stump must also be removed if the disease is to be eradicated. The apex of the pouch is then sutured to the anus about 1 cm above the dentate line and forms a reservoir for faeces. A loop ileostomy is raised to allow the extensive anastomosis to heal without contamination. Once the suture lines are healed the ileostomy is closed. The patient achieves continence since the anal sphincters remain intact. Patients who are severely ill at the time of original surgery can be treated initially by a colectomy with ileostomy. The rectal stump and sphincter are left *in situ* and a reservoir operation can be considered at a later date.[30]

This procedure avoids the patient having a permanent ileostomy but is a more complicated operation than proctocolectomy with permanent ileostomy. Careful selection of patients is, therefore, essential as several months may elapse between the original surgery and closure of the ileostomy.[30]

CRITERIA FOR CHOICE OF PATIENT

- Firm diagnosis of ulcerative colitis or familial polyposis coli.
- Both patient and partner must fully understand procedure and be aware of alternatives.
- Both patient and partner must be strongly motivated.
- The patient should have a stable emotional background.
- The patient must understand the time span for surgery.
- The patient should be under 50 years of age.
- The patient must have demonstrably competent anal sphincters.

URINARY RESERVOIRS

Methods of creating a continent urinary reservoir which can be emptied by self-catheterization are being researched. Among these are ileocaecal reservoirs and ileal pouches into which the ureters are implanted. Continence is achieved either by fashioning a nipple valve or relying upon the ileocaecal valve.[31] These procedures would facilitate appliance-free urinary diversion. Research into other possible methods of achieving urinary continence following diversion include the use of biocarbon spouts and subcutaneous magnets.

REFERENCES

1. Miles, W.E. (1908) A method of performing abdominoperineal excision for carcinoma of the rectum and of the terminal portion of the pelvic colon. *Lancet, ii*, 1812.
2. Waxman, B.P. (1983) Large bowel anastomoses: the circular staplers. *British Journal of Surgery. 70*, 64–77.
3. Heald, R.J. (1980) Towards fewer colostomies—the impact of circular stapling devices on the surgery of rectal cancer in a district hospital. *British Journal of Surgery, 67*, 198–200.
4. Hartmann, H. (1923) *Congrès Français de Chirurgie, 30*, 411.

5. Mittal, V.K., & Cortez, J.A. (1981) Hartmann procedure reconstruction with EEA stapler. In *Diseases of Colon and Rectum*, Ed. Goligher, J.C. Chap. 24, pp 215–6. London: Baillière Tindall.

6. Devine, H. (1937) Excision of the rectum. *British Journal of Surgery, 25*, 351.

7. Miller, G.G., Gardner, C.McG., Ribstein, C.B. (1949) Primary resection of the colon in ulcerative colitis. *Canadian Medical Association Journal, 60*, 584–5.

8. Brooke, B.N. (1952) The management of an ileostomy including its complications. *Lancet, ii*, 102–4.

9. Devlin, H.B. (1982) Stoma therapy review. In *Coloproctology*, No. 2, pp 8–16

10. Jenkinson, L.R., Houghton, P.W., Steele, K.V., Donaldson, L.A., & Crumplin, M.K.H. (1984) The Biethium Bridge—an advantage in stoma care. *Annals of Royal College of Surgeons of England. 66*, 420–2.

11. Nasmyth, D.G., Williams, N.S., Jones, D. & Smith, A.H. (1984) Comparison of defunctioning stomas: a prospective controlled trial. *British Journal of Surgery, 71*, 909.

12. Raimes, S.A., Mathew, V.V., & Devlin, H.B. (1984) Temporary loop ileostomy. *Journal of the Royal Society of Medicine, 77*, 738–741.

13. Morin, J.M. (1985) Urinary undiversion. *Journal of Enterostomal Therapy, 12*, 125–127.

14. Hendry, W.F. (1982) Urinary stomas part 1: surgical procedures and complications. *Clinics in Gastroenterology, 11*, No 2. 303–317.

15. Wallace, D.M. (1970) Uretero-ileostomy. *British Journal of Urology, 42*, 529–534.

16. Clarke, P.B. (1979) End-to-end ureteroileal anastomosis for ileal conduits. *British Journal of Urology, 51*, 105–109.

17. Heald, R. (1980) A staple in time saves a stoma. *Nursing Mirror* (3 January) 30–32.

18. Gillen, P., & Peel, A.L.G. (1986) A comparison of the mortality, morbidity and incidence of local recurrence in patients with rectal cancer treated by either stapled anterior resection or abdomino-perineal resection. In press.

19. Gillen, P., & Peel, A.L.G. (1985) Stapled anastomosis after anterior resection of rectum: which patients are at risk from anastomotic leak and local recurrence? *Coloproctology, 4*, 220.

20. Parrot, N. & Devlin, H.B. (1969) An alternative to colostomy. *British Medical Journal, i*, 6178.

21. Williams, N.S., & Johnson, D. (1983) The quality of life after rectal excision for low rectal cancer. *British Journal of Surgery, 70*, 460–462.

22. Devlin, H.B. (1982) Stoma therapy review. *Coloproctology, 3*, 18–26.

23. Goligher, J.C. (1984) Ulcerative colitis. *Surgery of the Anus Rectum and Colon*, 5th edn. Chap. 22, pp 805–970. London: Baillière Tindall.

24. Aylett, S.O. (1963) Ulcerative colitis treated by total colectomy and ileo rectal anastomosis: a ten year review. *Proceedings of the Royal Society of Medicine, 56*, 183.

25. Goligher, J.C. (1961) Surgical treatment of ulcerative colitis. *British Medical Journal, i*, 151.

26. Baker, W.N.W., Glass, R.E., Ritchie, J.K., & Aylett, S.O. (1978) Cancer of the rectum colectomy and colorectal anastomosis for ulcerative colitis. *British Journal of Surgery, 65*, 862.

27. Kock, N.G. (1969) Intra-abdominal reservoir in patients with permanent ileostomy. *Archives of Surgery, 99*, 223–231.

28. Palselius, I. (1982) Stoma care in continent ileostomy. *Clinics in Gastroenterology, 11*, No. 2, 278–284.

29. Parks, A.G., Nicholls, R.J. & Belleveau, P. (1980) Proctocolectomy with ileal reservoir and anal anastomosis. *British Journal of Surgery, 67*, 533–538.
30. Nicholls, R.J. (1983) Proctocolectomy: avoiding an ileostomy. *Nursing Mirror*, (16 February) 46–47.
31. Handley Ashken, M. (1982) *Urinary Reservoirs: Urinary Diversion.* Chap. 6, pp 112–140. London: Springer Verlag.

4 Selection and use of stoma care appliances

Early stoma appliances (Fig. 28) date back to the late 1700s when a French surgeon, Daguesceau, designed a leather pouch to collect body waste. Most patients, however, relied upon cups stuffed with cotton wool or dressings to absorb stoma effluent. Some more resourceful individuals improvised with household items such as empty tins and invented their own ingenious collecting devices.[1] In 1944 Koenig introduced a rubber bag.[2] This appliance represented a vast improvement for those coping with a stoma and some patients still prefer to use rubber bags today.

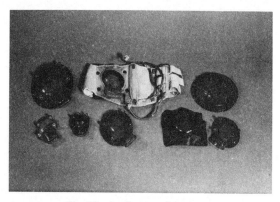

Fig. 28. *Appliances of yesteryear.*

Now an extensive choice of stoma care appliances is available. Many are disposable and incorporate hypoallergenic skin protective barriers. Most are made from soft odour-proof plastic, which is quiet and discreet. These appliances have significantly improved the quality of life for stoma patients. The vast selection of products and equipment available makes it easier for the nurse to meet the needs of individual patients. However, some nurses find it difficult to sort through such an array of products and identify a suitable appliance. The following information is intended as a broad guide to selecting the products that will best meet the needs of the patient.

TYPES OF STOMA APPLIANCE

There are basically three main types of stoma appliance: (Fig. 29)

1. *Closed bags:* Suitable only for end, iliac, or sigmoid colostomy when the motions are formed. If this appliance is suitable the patient should not need to change it more than once each day, twice at the very most.

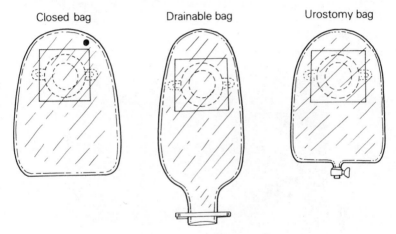

Fig. 29. *Three types of stoma appliance.*

2. *Drainable bags:* Suitable for semi-formed and fluid faeces, e.g. in the postoperative period and for transverse colostomy, ileostomy, and fistulae. The bag can be emptied as often as necessary as the bottom of the appliance is secured with a clip or tag. The frequency of changing varies depending upon the specific product.
3. *Urostomy bags:* Suitable for urine and the fluid effluent from high enterocutaneous fistulae. Most types incorporate a non-return valve to prevent the fluid splashing back up onto the stoma and a tap outlet for emptying. The frequency of changing varies depending upon the specific product. Most urostomy appliances have a facility to attach a 'night drainage' system.

The appliances can be further divided into two groups: one piece and two piece systems.

One-piece system

As the name suggests the appliance incorporates a method of securing the bag to the abdomen. This is usually an area of skin protective, such as a Karaya, carboxymethylcellulose or gum ring, and an area of hypoallergenic adhesive tape. Some appliances, however, feature a suitable area of skin protective only, which facilitates the bag adhering to the skin securely. Some feature only a small area of skin protective and are held in place by a belt. Others feature an area of hypoallergenic adhesive only, which is very flexible. The complete appliance is discarded after use and replaced with a new one.

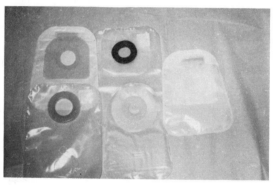

Fig. 30. *One-piece appliances.*

One-piece appliances usually have a precut opening to fit over the stoma, which is invariably round. It is imperative to select the correct gasket size. Careful measuring will indicate the correct size to fit snugly around the stoma, protecting all the surrounding skin. The opening must not be too small as this can cause constriction of the stoma and ischaemia can occur.

One-piece appliances are usually the most simple to apply and for this reason may be particularly suitable for patients with reduced manual dexterity, the elderly, or new patients, as less learning stages are required. They are available in closed, drainable, and urostomy types in a range of sizes. Specific details vary between products. (See Fig. 30.)

Two-piece system

These appliances consist of some sort of skin protective base plate or flange which adheres to the skin. The bags are then clipped or stuck onto this base. Some base plates are wafers of carboxymethylcellulose while others have a central area of skin protective surrounded by a hypoallergenic adhesive tape which usually proves to be more flexible. The base plate has to be cut out by the user and can be individually tailored to fit the stoma exactly. It is imperative that the base plate is cut out accurately and a cutting pattern should be used so that the correct fit is achieved. While it is fairly quick and simple to change the bag, some patients find the preparation process complicated. Cutting devices are available that will punch out an accurate opening. One appliance distribution company will precut flanges ordered from them on prescription if a cutting pattern is enclosed.[3]

The bags can be changed regularly and the base plate remains in position for several days depending upon the specific product. Two-piece appliances have the advantage that they can be cut to fit the stoma no matter what its shape. The bag can be changed without disturbing the surrounding skin, hence there is a lower incidence of skin irritation associated with its use.[1] Small bags can also be fitted when discretion is more important than capacity, e.g. for swimming, intimate occasions, and so on. Two-piece appliances are available in closed, drainable, and urostomy types in a range of sizes. Specific details vary between products. (See Fig. 31.)

Larger stoma appliances are also available and these are

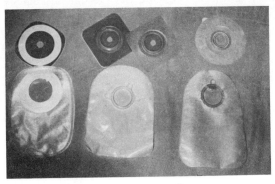

Fig. 31. *Two-piece appliances.*

particularly suitable when dealing with fistulae or bulky transverse colostomies. Almost all modern, disposable stoma care appliances are made from odour-proof laminated plastic. Most manufacturers produce appliances in a choice of clear or opaque material.

Clear plastic

These allow the stoma and effluent to be easily inspected and should always be used postoperatively. Some patients prefer to continue using a clear appliance as they find it easier to position the appliance accurately.

Opaque plastic

This may be tinted white or flesh-toned and is suitable for use when inspection is no longer required. Many patients prefer an opaque appliance since the bag's contents are disguised.

Flatus patches

These allow flatus to escape slowly via a puncture hole in the bag through an activated charcoal filter designed to absorb odour. These are integral on many closed appliances or may be fitted separately by the user. Flatus patches are available separately from some manufacturers' for use on appliances where none are supplied.

Appliances that 'balloon' due to flatus can be embarrassing. Flatus can be allowed to escape from drainable bags by opening the clip—this is only possible if privacy is available. Some patients dislike flatus patches and claim there is an odour despite the charcoal, or that they become clogged by liquid faeces. The filter should be attached to the bag in the top corner away from the area where faeces enter.

It is important to remember that the effectiveness of a charcoal filter is usually compromised after about 24 hours of use.

Pouch covers

These are available from most manufacturers, tailored to fit their appliance. These reduce sweating caused when plastic is in contact with skin and disguise the contents of the bag. Some are cotton and reusable, while others are disposable. One or two appliances feature a woven backing to prevent sweating and do not need to be covered.

ACCESSORIES

Skin protective wafers

There are several types of skin protective wafer available. These can be used to protect the skin around a stoma or fistula, having previously been cut accurately to the correct shape using a template. They all adhere to moist skin and allow healing to take place beneath them. Some are more flexible than others and most types are available in at least two sizes, e.g. $100\,mm^2$ and $200\,mm^2$. Some of these skin barriers are also available as rings or washers.

Filler pastes

These are invaluable for filling creases and crevices around a stoma or fistula, rendering the surface level for the attachment of a protective wafer or an appliance. They should be applied in thin layers and moulded with *damp* fingers. The layers can be built up until the correct level is achieved.

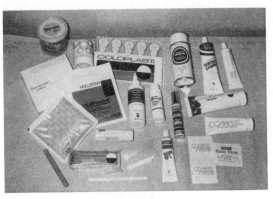

Fig. 32. *A selection of stoma care accessories.*

Protective powders

These will put a protective film on excoriated skin and also fill small crevices. They are powder preparations of the skin protectives.

Skin barriers

These are preparations that are applied to the skin as a protective layer to prevent damage occurring. Some create a plastic-type film on the skin while others dry, leaving an unnoticeable protective layer. All are non-greasy and do not compromise the adhesion of appliances. Some of these barriers make it easier to remove the appliance and thus reduce discomfort during bag changing. These products may be used therapeutically or prophylactically.

Deodorants

Deodorants are available to go inside the appliance to help to mask odours and kill odour-producing bacteria. Powder is available that is instilled into the bag and absorbs odours efficiently by a special oxidation process, although the powder itself has no smell. Small pocket-size air freshening atomizers are very useful for patients when they are dealing with their appliance away from home. However, it should be noted that there should not be any odour apparent if the patient is wearing a correctly fitted, modern appliance and leakage does not occur. There should only be an odour when the appliance is emptied or changed.

Stoma caps

These are small patches or mini-bags that cover the stoma but have minimal or no faecal capacity. They usually incorporate a flatus filter and are designed to be used by patients who control their colostomy by irrigation. They can also be very useful for swimming (and can be used for up to 30 minutes), for ileostomy patients and for covering a mucus fistula if the rectum remains *in situ*.

Stoma corsets

These are girdles made to measure by specialist manufacturers for stoma patients. A hole is incorporated to accommodate the stoma so that the patient has support without any pressure being exerted on the stoma. They are available with suspenders or as a pantie-girdle. Patients with a stoma are entitled to two corsets annually from the NHS, prescribable free of charge.

SELECTING AN APPLIANCE FOR AN INDIVIDUAL PATIENT

The majority of nurses will make a joint decision with the patient on a suitable product that meets his individual needs. Devlin emphasizes: 'The provision of a satisfactory appliance is essential to the ostomate, not only for physical but also for psychological reasons.'[4] The choice will be strongly influenced by the type and site of the stoma, the nature of the effluent and the patient's personal preference.

Points to consider

Postoperative appliances

- These must be of clear plastic to facilitate observation.
- They must be drainable as bowel motion is usually loose during the postoperative period.
- They may need to accommodate a support bridge, rod or ureteric catheter.
- They should protect skin around a stoma.
- They should be easy to apply and cause no discomfort.
- They should have a secure clip which is easy to use.
- They should be cosmetically acceptable.

Long-term use

Consider the patient's lifestyle, ability (physical and mental), employment, and hobbies with regard to the suitability of an appliance that is to be used long-term.

Consider which is suitable/preferable for the individual patient

- One-piece or two-piece?
- Clear plastic or opaque plastic?
- Skin protective only, skin protective and adhesive, or adhesive only?
- With a belt or without a belt?

Nursing observations

These should include the following observations of the patient:

- Physique.
- Position of stoma.
- Any complication, e.g. hernia.
- Type of skin.
- Manual dexterity.
- Mental ability.
- Shape and size of stoma.
- Nature of motions.
- What capacity is required.

Is it possible to accommodate patient's preferences in view of nursing observations? The patient must have a reliable, comfortable, and correctly fitted unobtrusive odour-proof appliance which does not leak or cause skin problems. The patient must have confidence in his/her appliance and, wherever possible, be able to complete a change without any aid to ensure independence.

Considerations when assessing appliances

Nurses are frequently shown appliances by representatives from the manufacturing companies. When assessing an appliance it may be helpful if the nurse applies the following questions:

1. Is it of good quality, well-manufactured from sound materials?
2. Is it made from plastic that incorporates an effective odour barrier (e.g. polyvinyldichloride)?
3. Is it quiet? Does it rustle?

4. Is it available in clear and opaque plastic?
5. Is it unobtrusive?
6. Does it incorporate a skin protective?
7. What is the adhesive like? Is it aggressive? Is it occlusive or microporous?
8. Is there a full range of gasket sizes available?
9. If it is a two-piece system, how does it fit together? Is this secure? Is it easy to accomplish?
10. If it is drainable, what type of clip is supplied? Is it secure? Is it easy to use? Is it discreet or bulky?
11. If there is a urostomy, what type of tap is incorporated?
12. Will the appliance attach securely to the skin?
13. Are there any rough edges or corners that could damage the stoma or skin?
14. Is there a flatus filter supplied? Does this appear effective? Is it integral or separate?
15. What advantages and benefits does it offer over my existing stock?
16. Which patient groups is it suitable for?
17. How much does it cost? How does that compare with similar products? Is it cost-effective?
18. How many must I order?
19. Will the manufacturer supply me with adequate samples to assess and try before I purchase?
20. What back-up services and support does the manufacturer offer?
21. How long does delivery take?
22. Are adequate stocks available to meet demand, i.e. will patients get supplies easily in the community?
23. Will patients be able to have confidence in it?
24. Would I wear it?

Nurses may come up against all manner of commercial pressure to induce them to use the products of a particular manufacturer.[5] The Royal College of Nursing has published the DHSS Draft Health notice *Acceptance of Funding, Gifts and Hospitality*. This should serve to make nurses aware of the possible implications of some commercial activities. If in any doubt, the nurse would be wise to seek advice from the nurse manager. If nurses are asked to conduct clinical trials or participate in market research they should proceed with caution, and should ensure that they are aware of the ethics relating to research and must respect the rules of confidentiality. Benefit may be had from seeking advice from the Health District's Ethical Committee if in any doubt.

Budgeting. The cost of stoma care appliances is a cause of concern to the DHSS purchasing authorities.[4] Most stoma care nurses have an influential role in advising nurse managers on budgets concerned with stoma appliances, as Fleming describes: 'The wise manager will refer to her on stock maintenance, prices and commonly used sizes and products.'[6] It is often a false economy to select only from a limited range of the cheapest products since this restricts the patient's choice and is more likely to result in product failure. This is distressing for the patient, more appliances are used, and skin problems that require treatment may result.

If the nurse is given budgeting responsibility for stoma care equipment, stock should be maintained cost-effectively and obsolescence avoided, bearing in mind that some appliances have a very limited shelf-life. One effective method is to establish a working capital of stock and to order on a topping-up basis. Thus only those products that have actually been used are replaced. New products can be included in the stock after adequate assessment. This may necessitate an older, less used product being deleted from the stock list.

BASIC PROCEDURE TO CHANGE AN APPLIANCE

1. Collect together all equipment, i.e: appliance; measuring guide; tissues (kitchen paper); accessories; warm water; disposal bag.
2. Prepare the new appliance, e.g. fit the clip, apply the flatus patch, instil deodorising powder, cut the flange.
3. Empty the appliance (if drainable).
4. Peel the appliance gently away from the skin from the top, support surrounding skin with the free hand.
5. Cover the stoma with tissue.
6. Wash peristomal skin with plain warm water and tissues, ensure all faeces is removed.
7. Dry skin thoroughly with tissues.
8. Apply skin protective, if used.

9. Measure the stoma to ensure that the appliance is the correct size.
10. Fit the appliance according to manufacturer's instructions, ensuring that the stoma is centrally placed in the opening.
11. Fit accessories, e.g. a belt or tape.
12. Check that the appliance and closure are secure and comfortable.
13. Wrap all soiled items in paper and dispose in refuse (closed bags may be emptied by cutting off the bottom of the bag prior to disposal).

REFERENCES

1. Cunningham, S.C. (1984) The cosmetics of stoma care. *Nursing, 30*, 890–895.
2. Strauss, A.A. & Strauss, S.F. (1944) Surgical treatment of ulcerative colitis. *Surgical Clinic of North America, 24*, 211–224.
3. Fittleworth Medical Ltd.
4. Devlin, H.B. (1985) Living with a stoma. In *Stoma Care To-Day*, Medicine Publishing Foundation pp 34–37.
5. Gardner, J.H. (1983) Commercial attention: a nurse's dilemma. *Stoma Care News, 3*, 9.
6. Fleming, J. (1984) Bags of choice. *Senior Nurse, 1*, (5 September), 13–17.

5 Psychological considerations in stoma care

Many patients who have undergone surgery resulting in a stoma will experience psychological disorders.[1] These may include:

- *Disturbance in body image*—the way the person saw himself before surgery is no longer an accurate picture.
- *Low self-esteem*—the stoma patient may believe himself now to be a 'lesser person'.
- *Poor self-concept*—the patient may no longer perceive himself to be 'a normal person'.
- *Obsessionalism*—the patient may become overfastidious and preoccupied with cleanliness.
- *Denial* (this is often an initial reaction after surgery)—the patient does not want to acknowledge what has taken place and is reluctant to look at the stoma.
- *Phantom rectum*—a feeling of still wanting to defecate after excision of the rectum, which may be associated with denial.
- *Repression*—the patient may subconsciously exclude the knowledge that he has a stoma or any information regarding the stoma.
- *Psychosocial problems*—the patient may be reluctant to go out and meet friends, go to work, or resume hobbies and activities due to a fear of rejection or of leakage and odour.
- *Psychosexual problems*—the patient may feel that he is no longer attractive to the opposite sex, or his own self-perception may be such as to make him unable to resume a sexual relationship.

These psychological responses to having a stoma can lead to depression, psychosis, and even suicide.[1] To help understand how some of these responses evolve it is necessary to look at some basic human psychological principles:

1. Psychological needs.
2. Psychological defence mechanisms.

3. Body image.
4. Self-perception.

PSYCHOLOGICAL NEEDS

What is a need?

According to Gillis: 'A need can be defined as a condition marked by a feeling of *lack* or *want* which requires the supply of a particular thing in order to be relieved.'[2] For example, if we are hungry we experience a feeling of 'want' which requires us to eat in order that the symptom is relieved. James defines it thus: 'A need is any deficiency whether physiological, e.g. food, or psychological, e.g. social acceptance.'[3]

Human needs can be split into two basic categories:

1. Basic or primary needs.
2. Secondary needs.

Primary needs

Primary needs are biological, the instincts of self-preservation, they are *inborn, universal,* and *eradicable.* They are the physiological and security needs. Abraham Maslow describes a hierarchy of needs which act as a motivation to human behaviour.[4] He describes primary needs as being:

1. Food ⎫
2. Water ⎬ Physiological
3. Oxygen ⎭
4. Warmth ⎫ Security
5. Reproduction ⎭

The remaining needs are psychological but also motivate and influence behaviour. Man is a highly developed being and his psychological needs are therefore very complex. Individuals develop a *drive* to satisfy their needs, i.e. the body will automatically strive to maintain a balance. A drive will not subside until the need is met. This process is known as *homeostasis.* If an individual's psychological needs are not met, the person will not stop wanting but will experience unpleasant emotions, which may manifest themselves in various ways depending upon the personality of the individual, e.g: depression; jealousy; tenseness; anger. These sensations will act as a drive to the individual to find alternative means of gratification.

Homeostasis

A deficiency is experienced
↓
Drive
↓
i.e. Individual strives to satisfy need
↓
Needs are satisfied
↓
Psychological well-being

If a need is not satisfied
↓
A deficiency is experienced
↓
Drive
↓
i.e. Individual strives to satisfy need
↓
Need is not satisfied
↓
Unpleasant emotion, e.g. frustration
↓
Drive
↓
i.e. Individual seeks alternative gratification

In understanding human needs and being aware of how a drive may be displayed the nurse is able to give help and support to the patient and his family. An understanding of needs can also be used to shape the patient's rehabilitation and can be used as a means of motivation.

Some human psychological needs are:

● Security.
● Social needs.

- Self-esteem, ego.
- Self-fulfilment.
- Recognition and respect.
- Interest and independence.
- Love.
- Friendship.
- Acceptance.

When considering these needs in relation to the patient having a stoma, two main factors are influencing the patient: the psychological effects of illness and hospitalization; and the change in body image and function.

Security needs

Altschul describes security thus: 'Security means the ability to predict what is going to happen and how to make things happen.'[5] When a patient is admitted to hospital, he often knows nothing of what is to happen, he is unsure of what is expected of him, and is often among strangers and in an alien environment. These factors will manifest into a feeling of insecurity. In the case of a stoma patient who is also unsure of what his future will be like with a change in the habits of a lifetime with regard to the elimination of body waste the insecurity is even greater. The patient is not able to predict what is going to happen and how to make things happen.

The patient is in need of information to satisfy his need for security, allowing him a full understanding of the situation. The nurse should acquaint the patient with the geography of the ward and explain ward routine; this will help him to feel more at ease in his surroundings. The patient should also be kept informed of what is going to happen to him, when, and also what is expected of him.

The nurse can build a strong link with her patient and this can aid security if the patient feels that he has someone with whom he can identify. Meeting the patient prior to admission can help alleviate insecurity by forming a familial link. Due to anxiety, the patient may retain little of the information he is given, and this will only add to his insecurity. The nurse should offer information gradually, as the patient is ready to accept it. A booklet or leaflet may prove helpful to aid the memory and allow the patient to read again the information he has been given.

Once the patient is able to feel in control of his situation and is aware of what is going to happen his need for security is more likely to be satisfied. The fact that the patient is no longer able to control his bowel function can leave his need to be in control unsatisfied and he will need time to adjust to this fact.

Social needs

In the words of Davis: 'The customs of the group to which we belong, influence behaviour produced to satisfy social needs to a very great extent.'[6] Human beings need to be part of a group and in all areas 'like' form into groups, e.g. the family group, trade unions, social clubs, and so on. When a patient is admitted to hospital he has a need to fit in. This can be helped by putting all newly admitted patients together and making introductions to other patients.

The stoma patient will worry about whether he can fit in if he feels that he is different from the group. He will need reassurance regarding his normality. Meeting another stoma patient with positive attitudes can help. The patient may also be anxious as to how the groups with whom he already identifies will react to him following his surgery, e.g. family, workmates, friends. The nurse will have to give the patient support and encouragement to resume his previous social activities after his operation. Introduction to the appropriate 'stoma association' may also prove advantageous in meeting the patient's need to fit in and feel part of the group.

Self-esteem needs

Recognition and respect. 'People like to feel they have a purpose in life. They have needs of attainment and recognition. This generates a drive towards status.' Human beings need to be appreciated, loved and thought well of in addition to feeling useful to others.

Immediately postoperatively the patient may feel he is a burden to the nurse who is dealing with his bodily function, which he has previously coped with alone and in private. He may find this degrading and thus the nurse must preserve the patient's dignity and show her respect for him to help preserve his self-esteem. As soon as it is practical the nurse should begin teaching the patient to deal with his own appliance and care for his stoma. Once he is learning, this can satisfy a need for attainment. Once he is competent enough to carry out the care of his stoma this will enable him to be independent and restore his status.

The patient may be anxious about his family's welfare, particularly if he is the breadwinner with dependants. He will probably have previously enjoyed recognition as the provider and will be eager to resume his responsibilities. Doubts about his capability may produce uncertainty about his future status. Will he be able to resume his job? How long will he be off work? The patient will need reassurance about his ability to work or advice and support regarding retraining. As soon as possible, the patient should resume his role in the family. Counselling of the family may be needed to facilitate this so that the patient is not treated as an invalid. This need can also be exploited to achieve rehabilitation.

After being in hospital a patient may realize that he is dispensable at home or work and that other people can fill the gap. This can present doubts in the patient's mind regarding his need for status. Careful counselling coupled with discussion with the family and, possibly, the employer may help to restore a sense of purpose for the patient.

Re-enforcement of desired behaviour is important and gives the patient a sense of achievement. A well-adjusted stoma patient with a positive attitude can be invaluable in reassuring the new patient; this not only helps the new patient but also meets a need for recognition thus helping the visitor to feel helpful and respected.[8]

Love. Stoma patients are often anxious as to what the effect of them having an alteration in bodily function will be on their family, friends, and sexual partners. Sensitive counselling and discussion of these problems will be required. The patient should be encouraged to express his feelings. Practical suggestions with regard to sexual relationships may also be required. It may be helpful to ensure that the patient's partner/family are aware that the patient will be watching their reactions to him closely.

Independence. The ability to cope with his own stoma and appliances will help restore the patient's independence. However, it may take time for the patient to accept that he is now dependent upon a bag. Being able to deal with his own stoma will meet the need of the patient to be self-sufficient, thus he will not then feel a burden.

PSYCHOLOGICAL DEFENCE MECHANISMS

'There is comfort in pretending that what we cannot have is not worth having.' (Aesop, 6th Century BC.)

How often do you hear 'I didn't really want the job anyway' from an unsuccessful candidate, or 'It was too expensive and poor quality' from the shopper who misses a sale bargain? Freud said of psychological defence mechanisms:

> 'They protect against external events or against internal anxiety, arousing impulses by distorting reality in some way. Defence mechanisms do not alter the objective conditions of danger; they simply change the way the person thinks about it. They involve an element of "self-deception".'[7]

> 'Defence mechanisms are to be found in everyday behaviour of normal people. Used in moderation they increase satisfaction in living and are therefore helpful modes of adjustment.'[7]

> 'A mental defence mechanism is an unconscious technique for reconciling a conflict.'[10]

There are many definitions of mental defence mechanisms, such as those above. They are ways of dealing with anxiety in the mind and may take several forms. The process takes place *unconsciously*.

'Ego defence' can be described: 'Whenever some cherished value is severely threatened some defence mechanism is brought into play. The new threatening information may be *denied*, or the thoughts and impulses stimulated by it may be *repressed*. Anger and hostility may be *projected* upon another source.'

In addition to the three common defence mechanisms mentioned here, there are several others. A patient who is to face life with a stoma may see his 'normal' bodily function as 'cherished' and now 'severely threatened', and so may employ defence mechanisms to enable him to deal with the situation psychologically. 'These defence mechanisms act as a form of mental anaesthetic to "lessen the pain" caused by conflicts between what our sensations tell us we are and what we think we ought to be.'[10]

If a patient's sensations such as sight and touch tell him that he has a stoma and that faeces are expelled from his abdomen into a bag while he thinks he ought to defecate normally via his anus this will produce a mental conflict. The nurse should be aware of the mental defence mechanisms the patient may employ in order to understand the reactions she may meet when dealing with the patient. These defence mechanisms are purely unconscious so the patient will not be aware of them. James describes the possible reactions: 'How an individual responds to a conflicting situation depends upon the individual (his past experience, his attitude and his motives), the nature and seriousness of the conflict and the environment which he is in.'[10]

Types of mental defence mechanism

Some mechanisms involve substitution

If a patient is met with a situation that he finds difficult and he is not able to improve his performance in a task to reach his personal ideal, he may feel inadequate. If he redirects his effort towards an activity where he has previously been successful he will probably perform this task very well. For example, if a patient finds that he cannot manage to change the flange of his appliance successfully he may feel inadequate. However, he may be able to apply a new bag to the flange easily so will turn his effort to this task and excel at it. The nurse will then find that the patient is reluctant to learn to change the flange despite being excellent at dealing with the bag. This is known as *compensation*. The patient may, however, redirect his effort away from care of his stoma and excel with his physiotherapy exercises, thus using a physical compensation.

Another defence mechanism similar to compensation is *sublimation*. Here the patient may try to find a goal that is more easily achieved than the one he finds difficult. If the nurse recognizes this and supplies a flange that he can apply more easily this will be more acceptable to the patient since he can attain his goal and satisfy his need for attainment.

Sublimation can also occur when psychological needs have to be repressed. The patient may impose unnecessary restrictions upon himself and find alternative goals to satisfy these. If the restrictions are unnecessary the nurse may be able to counsel the patient so that he can recognize this. For example, a young female patient may have strong maternal instincts but feel that a stoma may prevent her having children, and this may lead her to turn her maternal instinct towards a pet. Careful counselling and explanation may enable this patient to be aware that her maternal instincts can be satisfied. If such substitution takes place to an unhealthy degree it may become a perversion.

Another form of substitution is when the patient achieves his goal in his imagination, that is *day dreaming*. This is commonly seen in people who feel insecure or inferior and unable to cope; they can see no way out of their dilemma. Thus in their imagination they change the environment so that they can cope more successfully and the difference between 'actual self' and 'ideal self' is lessened.

Some mechanisms improve our chances of coping with our environment

There is a tendency to emulate others who are dealing with problems more successfully. This is not only conscious imitation but also occurs unconsciously, and it is known as *identification*. If the nurse introduces the patient to another with a stoma who is dealing well with similar problems it may allow identification to take place and the patient with the new stoma to emulate him. However, the nurse must ensure that the person with whom the patient identifies is a desirable model to follow.

Another common method of dealing with mental conflict is *regression*. Here the patient may resort to childish forms of behaviour which previously solved his problem by bringing attention and reassurance as well as physical help from his mother. This may take the form of crying, dependence, or a childlike attitude and conversation. The nurse should recognize these as the patient's call for help.

Some mechanisms convert mental anxiety into physical terms

These mechanisms may manifest in such activities as fiddling with clothes, biting nails, or wringing hands and can be recognized by the nurse as outward signs of inner anxiety. Others, such as smoking more heavily or eating excessively, may also occur. These are known as *compulsions*, e.g. compulsive eating.

A closely related mechanism is *psychosomatic illness*, which may have physical manifestations produced by anxiety. When the stoma nurse appears to teach the patient to change his bag he may complain of headache or nausea. This may be genuine, induced by his anxiety. The physical incapacity allows the patient to withdraw from a situation in which he feels that he will be unsuccessful without loss of face and is known as *conversion hysteria*.

A patient may be hostile towards the hospital team or towards himself and may deliberately (but unconsciously) create problems to deliver punishment, such as leaking bags or complaining of continually unsatisfactory care. An extreme of self-punishment is suicide. This form of problem-creating may be the patient's psychological call for help.

Some mechanisms ignore the existence of conflict

People can reject or forget experiences of which they do not wish to be reminded. They can actively forget and this is called *supression*, or unconsciously exclude the information, which is *repression*. This may render the patient unable to learn as he finds the experience of dealing with his stoma so unpleasant that he actively or unconsciously forgets what he has been told.

Repression may also manifest in other ways. If a patient's sexual desire is repressed because he feels his partner is repulsed by his stoma he may:

1. Become antagonistic towards anything that has sexual involvement. This is *reaction formation*.
2. Show an unhealthy interest in 'smutty talk' or pornography. This is *indirect expression of a repression*.

Another way of ignoring an experience that causes anxiety is *rationalization*. This is when information received by an individual about himself is interpreted as what he thinks it should be. To avoid this occurring the nurse must obtain feedback when dealing with the stoma patient. This will ensure that he has actually heard what has been said.

Patients may direct the 'blame' for their situation away from themselves, towards the surgeon, the nurse, or the family. This is *projection* and can cause hostile behaviour.

Some mechanisms avoid conflict by retreating from it

This may lead to the patient becoming very shy. He may avoid all social meeting and activities where he feels his shortcomings will be noticed by others. If this is recognized by the nurse she may be able to reassure the patient and rebuild his confidence to overcome this.

In summary, to quote James: 'Mental defence mechanisms are used by most people to some extent. In general, they are valuable anxiety-relieving techniques. However, in advanced cases a person may lose contact with reality and become psychotic.'[10] The nurse must be aware of these mechanisms when dealing with her patients, not only to enable her to understand their behaviour but also to recognize their inability or reluctance to learn. 'Because intense fear is an unpleasant emotion the defence mechanism may prevent the individual becoming aware of information of potential relevance. Negative attitudes may develop towards the source of relevant messages.' Hence the patient may develop a negative attitude towards the nurse whom he sees as 'the source of relevant messages'.

In a survey in 1950 among people with a high prejudice it was found that the intensity of the prejudice increased when attempts were made to present the disliked factor in a favourable light, and this finding too shows how the patient's capacity to learn and to accept the teacher (i.e. nurse) as a helper rather than a 'bearer of bad news' provoking hostile manners may be affected.

BODY IMAGE

The way we see ourselves (body image) plays an important part in our everyday lives. If there is a sudden alteration in this picture, e.g. after disfiguring surgery, it can have psychological implications on our behaviour. O'Brien describes body image as 'an intrapersonal experience of our feelings and attitudes towards our body and the way we organise our experiences'[12]; and Wilson explains: 'The body, its parts and functions have an individualised internal representation at any given moment; this "body image" is formed from birth by a group of visual perceptions, tactile explorations and sensations from other organs.'[11]

Body image provides a sense of existence and a basis of individual identity. It can also affect an individual's ability to perform. 'Skill in games and grace of movement are the result of accurate body image.'[13] Because a person has spent years developing his body image, the picture he has of himself will affect the way he feels about himself as a person. This will influence his interaction with other people. If a person has a mental image of his body that he feels is quite acceptable and 'normal' he will be able to interact with others in the usual social fashion. If, however, his body image is unacceptable to him, this will inhibit his interactions with others.

When an individual becomes ill he is often far more aware of his body. If this illness also involves a change in his body then he may have severe psychological difficulties coping with this alteration. The concept of body image is fluid and fragile, and if it is disrupted the patient may see himself as totally different after operation.[11] Sudden changes in a person's body image will, ultimately, produce psychological problems of acceptance. A change in long-standing body image cannot be suddenly accepted by the patient. A period of 'mourning' for the lost part may have to occur before the new image can be accepted.

Freud describes three stages of early development: oral, anal, and genital. In Freud's theory a child must master each stage successfully before moving on to the next aspect in order to develop a mature body image. The creation of a stoma changes a person's image of his body. Previously he has not been able to see his anus and has not had to actually handle or dispose of his body waste. In Western society children are often taught that body waste is 'dirty'. When a child is developing he may offer his body waste to his mother as a present, thinking of it as part of himself. This type of behaviour is discouraged and the subject of defecation is often taught to be taboo. When the patient in later life is faced with the situation of having an artificial anus on his abdomen and having to deal actively with his body waste this is contrary to his previous learning and requires a vast alteration in his body image.

Patients often take some time to adapt psychologically to this. Some experience the phenomenon of 'phantom rectum'. In some cases the patient knows his rectum has been removed but, because the psychological process has not adapted to the change in body image he may still feel the urge to defecate. However, phantom rectum may be an entirely physiological phenomenon.

When discrepancies occur in body image because of the

differences in the way a patient has always perceived his body and now because of his stoma the way he currently sees it, mental conflict will occur. This conflict can produce many anxieties which will manifest in various ways. The patient may fear rejection from friends and family; he may feel abnormal or a lesser person. Furthermore, a stoma not only alters the body's external physical appearance but also removes the ability to control elimination so this acts as a double assault on the body image.

As previously stated an individual's body image has a direct bearing on his interpersonal behaviour. In the case of the stoma patient whose body image has been suddenly altered, his interaction with others may also be affected. This may mean that he becomes socially isolated because he fears he is different. The extent to which disfiguring surgery affects body image can depend upon the age of the patient when the surgery takes place. For instance, a child who has not fully developed his body image would probably suffer little as he could incorporate the change into his developing image. In adolescence the individual is most preoccupied with attractiveness and normality and a change in body image at this age would be very psychologically traumatic. In the older age group, although appearances and normality have ceased to be of paramount importance the individual's body image has been established for a longer period of time, and so adjustment may be very difficult.

A patient who has experienced a change in body image will need much support and encouragement from the nurse. He may need continually to discuss his thoughts in order to come to terms with them. The nurse should enlist help from the patient's family to encourage acceptance.

SELF-PERCEPTION

The concept a person has of himself will influence his behaviour and opinion as it is part of his personality. Self-concept can influence the mental state of an individual and is responsible to some extent for our attitudes and mental well-being. As Sprott explains:

'When we think of a normal human being we think of a person who can walk and talk, reflect and reason and who is aware of himself as a person, thus rendering him capable of pride and shame, ambition and disappointment. Human beings vary in their capacity for reasoning, in the ideas they have about themselves and in their proneness to worry about the figure they are cutting.'[14]

All individuals have a conception of what they perceive as a 'normal person', and this conception will influence their opinion of themselves as a person and also their opinion on the normality of others. Infants are unable to comprehend themselves as individuals; the process is learned. This is a gradual awareness of oneself as a separate individual, which is influenced by development. Other characteristics will influence the self-concept such as appearance, physique, and social standing. These enable the individual to make a comparison between himself and others and also between himself and his idea of an ideal person. The characteristics that one person takes into account may not be the ones another individual will take his cues from. Such differences as sex and social class will influence an individual's self-conception.

The concept a person has of himself will influence his behaviour and opinion, it is part of his personality. Rogers describes a personality theory in which the most important concept is 'self'.[15]

'"The self" consists of all the ideas, values and perceptions that characterise the individual, what he is and what he can do and cannot do. The way a person sees himself will influence not only his behaviour but also the way he sees other people and the world in general. If a person has a positive self concept he will view the world around him in a different way to a person whose self concept is weak. The perceived self may not be a true image, e.g. a successful and highly respected business man may see himself as a failure.'

Self-concept has a strong influence on the individual's acceptance of situations and experiences. He will compare every experience with his self-concept and assess it. An individual always wants to behave in a way that is in keeping with his self-image. If he encounters a situation or feeling that is incompatible with his self-concept he will find it threatening and may deny its existence in conscious thought. The more areas a person finds that are not compatible with his self-concept the more the areas are repressed.

This leads to a wider division between the self and reality and will create anxiety. If a person's self-concept is consistent with his experience and behaviour then he will not have to repress many experiences and will be well balanced psychologically.

Rogers' personality theory also describes another self that he terms 'ideal self'. This is an individual's conception of the person he would like to be—his ideal. The concept a person holds as his ideal is an influence upon his personality, his behaviour, and his psychological state. If the ideal self is very similar to the individual's self-concept then he will be happy and fulfilled. If the difference between ideal-self and self-concept is great the person may be dissatisfied with himself as an individual and unhappy.

Thus individuals have to cope with two types of discrepancy with their self-concept, i.e. the difference between self-concept and reality, and the difference between self-concept and ideal self. The self-concept is very important to an individual's behaviour and can influence strongly his beliefs. Teenagers often experience hero-worship and attempt to imitate the person they hold as their ideal. They also have 'crushes' on people they feel they would like to emulate. When a patient has surgery which includes the creation of a stoma it is unlikely that he will be able to fit this easily into his self-concept. This is a reality, and the greater the difficulty the patient has accepting the change in body image and fitting into his self-concept, the greater the difficulty he will have accepting the stoma. A stoma is most unlikely to feature in an individual concept of ideal self and will, again, cause difficulty with acceptance.

As previously discussed, a person who is capable of fitting his experiences with self-concept is well adjusted; if this is no longer the case, he may well be psychologically disturbed. Similarly, if his self-concept and ideal self are now poles apart, he may feel very dissatisfied with himself as a person.

If a person holds a concept of himself as being 'normal' and 'acceptable' by others he will be able to function well socially. If this is changed suddenly, as with surgery for a stoma, he may well feel abnormal and unacceptable, fearing that he smells or that his stoma is detectable. This will inevitably alter his social interactions and habits and he may be socially isolated. In conclusion, the statement 'I am what I think I am' has much truth about it. An individual's self-conception has much influence upon his personality, and will influence his attitude and behaviour.

REFERENCES

1. Devlin, H.B., Plant, J.A., & Griffin, M. (1971) The aftermath of surgery for ano-rectal cancer. *British Medical Journal, iii*, 413.
2. Gillis, L. (1972) *Human behaviour in illness*, Chap. 2, p. 34. London: Faber and Faber.
3. James, D.E. (1975) *Introduction to Psychology*, Chap. 6, p.161. London: Panther.
4. Maslow, A.H. (1943) A theory of human motivation. *Psychology Review, 50*, 370.
5. Altschul, A. (1972) *Psychology for Nurses*, Chap. 9, p.106. London: Baillière Tindall.
6. Davis, A. (1943) Child training and social class. In *Child Behaviour and Development*. Ed. Barker, R.G. New York: McGraw-Hill pp.607–19.
7. Hillgard, E.R., Atkinson, R.B., Atkinson, R.L. (1975) *Introduction to Psychology*, Chap. 15, p. 442. New York: Harcourt Brace Jovanovitch.
8. Trainor, M.A. (1982) Self-help groups. Part 2. *Clinics in Gastroenterology, 11*, 415-419. London: Saunders.
9. International Ostomy Association Professional Advisory Pamphlet No. 2, 1981.
10. James, D.E. (1975) *Introduction to Psychology*, Chap. 5, p. 105. London: Panther.
11. Wilson, D. (1981) Changing the body's image. *Nursing Mirror*, 2 April, 38–40.
12. O'Brian, J. (1980) Mirror, mirror, why me? *Nursing Mirror*, 24 April, 36–37.
13. Altschul, A. (1972) *Psychology for Nurses*, Chap. 2, p.30. London: Baillière Tindall.
14. Sprott, W.J.H. (1958) *Human Groups*, Chap. 2, p. 23. Penguin.
15. Roger, C.R. (1959) A theory of therapy, personality and interpersonal relationships as developed in the client centred framework. In *Psychology—a Study of Science*, Vol. 13. Ed. Koch, S. New York: McGraw Hill. pp. 184–256.

6 Counselling

Communication between the nurse and patient is fundamental to all nursing care. Some nurses suggest that counselling should be an integral part of nursing practice.[1] There are several counselling models that will enable the counsellor to help his client come to terms with a problem, although specific detail is beyond the scope of this book. Much has been written on the subject and suggested further reading is listed at the end of this chapter.

Some nurses are frightened when talking to patients who are facing emotional problems in case they invoke a situation that they feel ill equipped to handle.[2] This may prompt the nurse to use avoidance tactics. Some nurses frequently counsel patients in the course of their work without necessarily recognizing it as such. In stoma care nursing counselling is an integral part of the nurse's role.

Patients who are undergoing surgery involving a stoma have to face many problems and uncertainties, which are discussed elsewhere in this book. If the surgery is being performed to remove a cancer there is the added uncertainty regarding prognosis; will the cancer recur? If so, when? It is important that we as nurses help these patients to explore their feeling towards their illness and surgery with a view to eliciting their specific problems and helping them come to terms with them. A recent research project involving patients who had a stoma for cancer of the bowel or bladder, indicated that supportive counselling resulted in a positive alteration in self-concept/self-esteem, enabling the patients to adapt more positively to their stoma.[3]

There are training courses for counselling available for nurses. Attendance at such a course can be extremely advantageous to nurses who are regularly in contact with stoma patients. The English National Board Clinical Courses in Stoma Care also devote a substantial proportion of the syllabus to counselling and communication skills. Nurses who undertake counselling regularly often find it quite stressful because they open themselves to the patient's pain. It is therefore essential that they, themselves, have support.

The successful nurse–counsellor must firstly be aware of herself as a person. 'One of the main stumbling blocks to effective counselling is an inability to come to terms with one's feelings.' 'In most cases feelings are quickly communicated from one person to another.'[1] It is essential to effective counselling that the nurse prevents her own attitudes, values, and prejudices from becoming apparent to the patient. The nurse must also recognize her own limitations and the need for referral to another professional if she realizes that the problem is beyond the scope of her expertise. Referral should take place with the patient's consent and the nurse must take care to ensure that the patient does not feel brushed aside or dismissed by the action. The reason for the referral should be explained and the nurse should not be afraid to admit that she does not have the necessary skills.

In formal counselling situations the counsellor meets with his client on a regular basis, usually weekly for a fixed period of time, perhaps one hour. However, in nursing this is often not a practical arrangement, thus most counselling takes place as and when the situation demands.

WHAT IS COUNSELLING?

The British Association for Counselling's definition states:

> 'Counselling is a process through which one person helps another by purposeful conversation in an understanding atmosphere. It seeks to establish a helping relationship in which the one counselled can express his thoughts and feelings in such a way as to clarify his own situation, come to terms with some new experience, see his difficulty more objectively and so face his problem with less anxiety and tension.'

> 'It provides the client with the opportunity to explore, discover and clarify ways of living more resourcefully and towards greater well-being.'

One way in which counselling fits into nursing is outlined by distinguishing four types of helping strategy.[4]

1. *Direct action:* Taking action yourself to provide for someone else's needs, e.g. changing an appliance for a patient.

2. *Giving advice:* Making suggestions about courses of action another person can and possibly should take, looking at it from your own position, e.g. advising a method of treating excoriated skin.
3. *Teaching:* Helping someone acquire the knowledge and skills you think they need, e.g. teaching the patient to change his own appliance.
4. *Counselling:* Helping someone explore a problem so they can decide what to do about it, e.g. enabling the patient to elicit the possible solutions to his problem and select the most suitable alternative.

'In counselling the emphasis is placed squarely on the other person involved, rather than on the helper.'[5]

Any counselling situation involves: a *counsellor* who is seeking to help another; a *client* who is seeking help; and a *problem*. The objective is to help the client to recognize and clarify his problem, finding his own resources to cope, thus enabling him to develop a greater knowledge of himself and others.

Throughout this Chapter I have used the title 'nurse' and 'patient' rather than 'counsellor' and 'client' as I feel it is more appropriate.

COUNSELLING AIMS AND OBJECTIVES

To facilitate effective counselling the nurse should endeavour to:

- Be genuine and natural.
- Create a conducive environment.
- Indicate that she has time.
- Show respect, build trust.
- Establish a rapport with the patient.
- Listen actively/be attentive.
- Give encouragement.
- Give feedback to the patient.
- Clarify what has been said and the meaning of particular words to the patient.
- Use open questions.
- Convey empathy.
- Observe non-verbal behaviour/body language.

The environment

To facilitate effective counselling it is important to create a conducive atmosphere. There should be privacy; ideally in hospital, counselling should take place in a separate room that is away from the general ward. If this is not possible then a degree of privacy can be achieved by screening the bed. A patient is unlikely to disclose his innermost anxieties in a public place with an inquisitive listener nearby. If there is a room set aside for counselling it should create an informal atmosphere with confortable chairs for the counsellor and client of a similar height, with no barrier such as a desk in between. Interruptions should be avoided as they can disrupt the helping process or may occur just as the patient is about to disclose his problem.

Time

Many patients stereotype nurses as busy. It is essential that the nurse conveys to the patient that she has time and is willing to listen to what he has to say. Sitting down with the patient rather than standing as if poised to rush off is important.

Respect

The nurse should endeavour to indicate to the patient that she respects him and sees him as a person of worth in his own right. She should indicate a desire to help him find a solution to his problem. The patient should feel that he has her undivided attention.

Establish rapport

It is important to establish a rapport with the patient and to strive towards a trusting relationship in which he feels able to disclose his anxieties. Very few people will feel able to voice personal problems to a stranger until they have established at least some rapport.

Listen

The ability to listen actively and interpret what the patient is saying is important. 'In counselling it is important to listen to what is said and also to listen to what is being implied by the words.'[6] In order to listen effectively the nurse must be attentive and not planning her next answer which may cause her to miss an important cue at the end of a sentence.[7] If she is preoccupied with other issues, is anxious, or has preconceived ideas about what is to be said this will inhibit effective listening.

Give encouragement

Once the patient has started to talk about his anxieties the nurse should encourage him to share his feelings with her. This may be a very painful process for the patient and the nurse should offer her support to facilitate disclosure. The patient may be fully aware of what his problem is but be unable to find an acceptable solution. In other cases a patient may have identified a particular problem area but be unable to clarify the specific aspect that concerns him most. Equally the nurse may wrongly assume that when a patient tells her about an area of anxiety she understands his specific problem. For example, the patient who confides 'It's my job that worries me' could mean any of the following:

1. 'I'm afraid the appliance will leak during my activities at work.'
2. 'My colleagues at work will shun me now that I've got a colostomy.'
3. 'I will not be able to go to work as there are no suitable facilities to cope with my appliance.'
4. 'Joe Smith has been waiting for an opportunity to step into my shoes for years, this period of sickness will give him the excuse he needs.'
5. 'There's a lot of redundancy where I work, a long period of sickness is sure to put my name on the list.'
6. 'They won't be able to cope at work if I'm not there.'

The nurses must, therefore, explore further to elicit exactly what the problem involves.

Give feedback

It is important to give the patient feedback to demonstrate that the nurse has actually heard what he has said. This also gives the nurse an opportunity to clarify that her understanding is, in fact, correct. 'So you are telling me that you are frightened to return to work in case the appliance leaks while you are with a customer?' This is called reflecting back and it is ideal to use the patient's own key words.

Clarify

It is also helpful to clarify exactly what the term the patient is using means to him, for instance to ask questions such as: 'What exactly does being frightened mean to you, how does it feel?' While it is essential to convey to the patient an acceptance of his situation and to endeavour to see the problem through his eyes the nurse must elicit what the patient perceives to be 'normal'. What one individual sees as an acceptable, everyday occurrence, another will identify as a crisis.

Open questions

Using open questions that cannot be answered with a simple 'yes' or 'no' encourages the patient to explore further, e.g. 'How do you feel about having a colostomy?' will give a much fuller insight into the patient's thoughts than 'Does having a colostomy worry you?'.

The nurse should avoid asking questions merely to collect information; counselling must not become an interrogation. It may be helpful to avoid using the word 'why' as this can sound more probing than 'what' or 'how'. For example: 'Why can't you return to work now you've got a colostomy?' will probably elicit a less meaningful reply than: 'What is it about having a colostomy that will stop you returning to work?' or 'How do you feel that having a colostomy will prevent you returning to work?'

Empathy

It is essential that the nurse conveys to the patient a feeling of empathy, which has been described as the ability to see the world through another person's eyes. 'Empathy is not sympathy; this is to be affected by the same feeling, a mental participation in another's trouble. Empathy is the power of projecting one's personality into the object of contemplation and so fully comprehending'.[8] Tschudin uses the example of the helper going to the aid of a person who has fallen into a ditch. She explains that the *sympathetic helper* goes and lies in the ditch with him and bewails the situation with him; the *unsympathetic helper* stands on the bank and shouts to the victim, 'Come on, get yourself out of that ditch'; and the *empathetic helper* climbs down to the victim but keeps one foot on the bank, thus being able to help the victim out of trouble onto firm ground again.[9] The nurse should try to demonstrate empathy with the patient by telling him his feelings are understood. 'Yes, I'm sure it can be very frightening to be going back to work after having a colostomy, I can understand your anxiety.' This conveys an acceptance of the patient's problem and may encourage him to talk more frankly.

The nurse should not be afraid of silences during counselling as they can be productive and facilitate collection of her thoughts. However, if silences become lengthy and uncomfortable the nurse may need to prompt the patient.

Body language

An awareness of body language can be helpful and the nurse should notice if the patient appears ill at ease or tense. He may fail to make eye contact, constantly shuffle in his chair, or physically withdraw, leaning away and folding his arms and legs. The nurse should endeavour to convey openness by establishing eye contact, smiling, sitting in a relaxed position, and appearing receptive. Touch can also be a means of communicating empathy and caring to the patient. Some patients will respond readily to a gesture such as resting a hand on the arm. The nurse must, however, judge each case separately as some individuals are uncomfortable with physical contact and shrink from it. (See Figs 33 and 34.)

EXPLORING SOLUTIONS

Once a specific problem has been identified the nurse can help the patient to explore the possible solutions. As previously stated

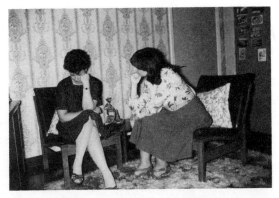

Fig. 33. *Patient ill at ease and tense.*

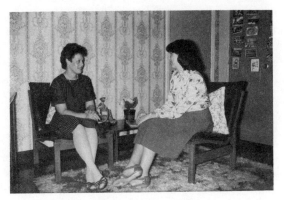

Fig. 34. *Conveying openness.*

counselling is not giving advice, thus a response such as 'I think the best thing for you to do is...' or 'If I were you I'd...' is totally inappropriate. A more suitable response would be, 'So your main fear is that the appliance will leak while you are with a customer. Let's look at the ways in which you can cope with this'. The nurse should then work through the various possible alternatives with the patient, discussing the feasibility and practicality of each. It can be recognized that there may be numerous alternatives, for example:

1. Devise a strategy to overcome the anxiety and create confidence in the appliance.
2. Avoid contact with customers.

3. Only have contact with customers immediately after appliance change.
4. Manage colostomy by irrigation thus avoiding the necessity of wearing an appliance.
5. Change job.
6. Retire from work.

This is quite a simple example but with a more complex problem involving interpersonal or sexual relationships the alternatives may be much more diverse. It is essential that the nurse guides the patient to select the solution which he feels is most suitable, as this has the greatest chance of success; what can appear to be an obvious and acceptable solution to the problem for the nurse may be totally unacceptable or out of character to the patient.

As nurses we are used to giving advice and 'telling'; in counselling this is a tendency that must be curbed. However, the patient will often expect the nurse to tell him what to do, and the nurse must then make it clear that while the problem cannot be solved for him, he or she will help him to find a way to solve it.

PLANNING AND ACHIEVING GOALS

Once a particular course of action has been decided upon the patient should be helped to plan his specific goals and look at ways in which these can be achieved. For example, if the patient who is frightened to return to work because of anxiety regarding appliance leakage decides that the most acceptable solution is to overcome his anxiety, his goal is to achieve confidence in his appliance. This may involve several stages and the nurse should help him to establish ways of attaining his objective, for example:

1. Trying various appliances and selecting the one he feels to be the most secure.
2. Wearing the appliance and gaining confidence in the company of close family or friends where, if a leakage occurs, it would be less devastating.
3. Increasing confidence in the appliance by going out and meeting strangers, e.g. shopping.
4. Building up confidence in the appliance by demonstrating its security at social functions.

5. Meeting with customers in groups or with a colleague which provides the opportunity to withdraw if the patient feels it to be necessary.
6. Meeting with customers on an individual basis.

Once a plan has been established and the method of achieving his goals agreed the patient should carry out the chosen method. He should formulate a time plan and discuss his progress with the nurse at future meetings. This will enable him to evaluate the success of his strategy and assess if the problem is resolved or more action needs to be taken.

It may not be possible for the nurse to meet with the patient following discharge but a valuable contribution will have been made if he can be helped to:

- Explore the situation and clarify what his actual problem is.
- Select an appropriate course of action.
- Set goals to achieve his solution.
- Evaluate whether his strategy has been successful.

William Stewart describes a counselling model likening these stages to the problem solving approach involved in the nursing process,[10] i.e:

1. Assessing and identifying the problem.
2. Planning the action to be taken.
3. Implementing the action.
4. Evaluating the outcome.

This can be a very useful comparison in helping the nurse structure her counselling, control the interview, and follow a logical progression.

DIFFICULT QUESTIONS

Sometimes patients ask questions which nurses find difficult to answer such as: 'It's cancer, nurse, isn't it?' In such a situation nurses may be reluctant to answer in case the patient becomes distressed and they are unable to cope. They might hesitate to answer due to anxiety about the response of the medical staff to such action.

If questions such as this are ignored, avoided, or the nurse lies, the patient may feel terribly frustrated, angry, or cheated and this

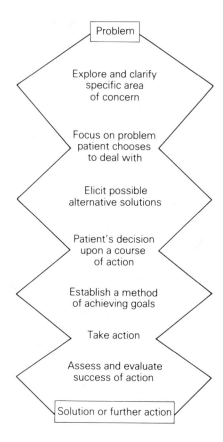

Fig. 35. *Basic counselling strategy.*

can be damaging to any trusting relationship that is developing between him and the nurse. It may also make it more difficult for the patient to cope. In this situation a helpful response may be, 'What makes you think that it's cancer?'. This gives the nurse a little time to collect her thoughts while the reply should enable a judgement to be made on whether the patient wants his statement confirmed or is looking for reassurance. If the nurse is sure that the patient is seeking information about his diagnosis then this should be given. Bad news should always be tempered with hope. However, it is essential to avoid premature or false reassurance.

The nurse should approach the situation with positive optimism, e.g. 'Yes it is cancer and I'm sure you must see that as very bad news. The good news is that your condition can be treated and doctor is very hopeful that you will make a full recovery'.

Some patients do not want to know they have cancer and cope with the situation by not acknowledging it (denial). If this is the case then the nurse should accept that it is the patient's way of coping with the situation, and should not challenge his denial. If the patient becomes very distressed or upset then the nurse should clarify the reason for this. Reassurance should not be given until the nurse has established what the patient is upset about and why. The nurse should aim to model the response to what the patient wants to know and should not force unwanted thoughts onto him or withhold information he is seeking.

SEXUAL COUNSELLING

Counselling to overcome problems encountered in their sexual relationships may be required by patients who have a stoma. Difficulties in sexual function may arise as a result of damaged tissues or distorted anatomy following surgery, (see Chapter 1) or psychological disturbance. The presence of a stoma results in altered body image and self-concept. If the patient considers himself unattractive to the opposite sex, or has fears of embarrassment or failure, this may result in diminishing libido in turn resulting in negative self-esteem.

Prior to undertaking sexual counselling the nurse should have certain competencies. Shipes and Lehr[11] suggest that these are:

1. Acceptance of and comfort with one's own sexuality and that of others.
2. Realization that one's sexuality and sexual expression are essential for self-esteem.
3. Awareness of one's own values regarding sex.
4. Knowledge of sexuality.
5. Ability to communicate with ease regarding sex.
6. Ability to accept where a patient is, at a given time, in relation to his sexuality.
7. Knowledge of when and where to refer.

An understanding of specific sexual problems together with their likely causes and treatments is an advantage. There are specific courses available for psychosexual counselling[12] which nurses involved with stoma patients may find advantageous.

According to Glover: 'In order to accept the sexuality of patients, the nurse must first accept her own sexuality.'[13] It is important that the nurse recognizes and accepts her own attitudes, values, and beliefs and is comfortable with them. If she is unaware of her reactions these may be transmitted to the patient via non-verbal messages and appear judgemental.[11] In sexual counselling it is essential to display acceptance and avoid moral judgement. The decision of which practices are acceptable and which must remain taboo can only be made by the partners within the relationship and not by anyone else. It is therefore important if the counselling is to be a decision-making process regarding actual sexual practices that the partner is also included; partner involvement in all aspects of sexual counselling is advantageous. The nurse must be at ease when discussing sexual activities. Any embarrassment or unease will be communicated to the patient who may then become tense.

Some words may carry a very negative connotation, e.g. 'inadequate', 'dysfunction', 'frigid', 'impotent', and 'incompetent'. These should be avoided and replaced with words such as 'concern' and 'dissatisfaction'.[11] It is also essential to use language and terminology that is familiar to the patient. It is pointless using anatomical nouns such as 'penis', 'vagina' or 'clitoris' or referring to activities such as 'sexual intercourse' or 'cunnilingus' if the patient has no conception of what is meant. If the patient is more familiar with colloquial terms then these are the words that should be used. The nurse must, however, establish that her understanding of the terms is correct since thingy or it can mean several things!

When talking to patients about their sexual concerns the nurse should avoid conveying the attitude that sex is wonderful and he should be enjoying it, because this may be inappropriate. It is important to determine what the patient's sex life was like before he had a stoma and ascertain what effect he perceives the stoma to have had. The nurse should try to establish how important sex is to the patient's lifestyle. Some patients who were disinterested in sex prior to surgery or who did not find it pleasurable may see the stoma as an ideal excuse, giving them a way out. If this is the case then the nurse should respect it and avoid pressing the issue.

Consideration must be given as to the patient's readiness to talk about his sexual concerns. The topic is often best introduced into general conversation once a rapport has been established. A question such as 'How do you feel that this operation has affected your relationship with your wife?', will provide the patient with an opportunity to broach the subject of sex if he feels ready, but if he does not feel able to disclose his sexual anxieties a non-specific answer is still appropriate. In some cases the nurse may judge it to be appropriate to ask a more direct question such as 'Many patients feel anxious about their sex life after having a stoma, how do you feel?'. This has the effect of giving the patient 'permission' to voice his doubts and fears about sex which he may have been reluctant to do, viewing it as a very private and personal aspect of his life. The nurse should create opportunities to explore sexual activity and potential problems without prying.

When discussing sexual activity it is wise to commence with the least threatening questions and observe the patient's response before broaching more intimate topics such as masturbation or oral sex which he may be ill at ease with, causing him to withdraw. Sexual counselling, like any other counselling, should focus on eliciting the actual problem and facilitating the patient finding his own solution. To do this the patient may require certain information and practical suggestions which are discussed in Chapter 17.

Some nurses feel ill at ease discussing sexual problems with patients and thus feel unable to undertake sexual counselling. If this is the case then the patient should be referred to a professional who has the relevant expertise to deal with the problem. It must be stressed that this referral must be handled with extreme sensitivity. The patient may have had to muster a lot of courage to enable him to voice his problems and a referral may appear to be a rebuff.

The Family Planning Association, Marriage Guidance Council, and Association for the Sexual and Personal Relationships of the Disabled (SPOD) all offer a counselling service to help patients overcome sexual problems. It is essential to explain to the patient that these organizations, despite their title, have a wider range of functions than merely birth control or dealing with marital disharmony.

WHAT SHOULD BE AVOIDED IN COUNSELLING?

1. The nurse should avoid doing too much talking, it should be the patient who ventilates and explores his problem with encouragement and prompting from the nurse.

2. The nurse should not criticize the patient in any way by word or gesture. She must avoid allowing her personal attitudes and beliefs to become apparent. Counselling does not involve registering approval or disapproval. No moral judgements should be made.

3. The nurse should not ask questions that can be answered with 'yes' or 'no' (closed questions), allowing the counselling situation to become an interrogation or opportunity for collecting irrelevant information.

4. The nurse should not use avoidance tactics, failing to allow the patient to explore his problem; if the approach is made by the patient at an inappropriate time, the problem should still be recognized and a promise made to help. For example, if a patient begins to voice his problem at a time when the nurse is unable to give him her full attention a response such as: 'I can understand that you will be worried about having a colostomy, I'll come back to you at 2 o'clock so that we can talk about the problems without me being interrupted.' This is a far more acceptable response than 'Cheer up, don't worry, I'm sure it will be all right in the end. Everybody feels a bit like that but they get over it sooner or later'.

5. The nurse should avoid befriending the patient. Although a counselling relationship is personal and based upon trust it should remain professional. The nurse should also avoid cultivating the patient's dependence.

6. Manipulation of the situation should be avoided; the nurse should attempt to provide the right conditions to facilitate purposeful conversation.

7. The nurse should avoid merely giving advice; the aim of the nurse in counselling is to help the patient seek his own solution. However, patients facing a crisis need directional counselling, whereas non-directive counselling is more suitable to decision making, that is the patient arguing with himself regarding his options.

8. The nurse should never appear bored, impatient, hostile, or patronizing. She should avoid interrupting or jumping to conclusions. Body gestures can be distracting, such as a particular mannerism or fiddling with something.

9. The nurse must avoid having preconceived ideas of what the problem will be and what it means to the patient. All patients

are individuals and even if a problem is familiar it may affect one patient in a totally different way to another.

FURTHER READING

Nurse, G. (1980) *Counselling and The Nurse: An Introduction.* Aylesbury: H.M. & M.
Tschudin, V. (1982) *Counselling Skills for Nurses.* London. Baillière Tindall.
Stewart, W. (1983) *Counselling in Nursing: A Problem Solving Approach.* London. Harper & Row.
Egan, G. (1982) *The Skilled Helper.* California: Brooks/Cole Publishers.
Kennedy, E. (1982) *On Becoming a Counsellor.* Dublin. Gill & MacMillan.
Shipes, E.A. & Lehr, S.T. (1980) *Sexual Counselling for Ostomates.* Springfield, Ill.: Charles C. Thomas.

REFERENCES

1. Bleazard, R. (1984) Knowing oneself. *Nursing Times.* 7 March, 44–46.
2. Maguire, P. (1983) Counselling. *Nursing Mirror.* 29 June, 60.
3. Watson, P.G. (1983) The effects of short-term post-operative counselling on cancer/ostomy patients. *Cancer Nursing*, February, 21–29.
4. Hopson, B. (1978) Counselling—a case for demystifying and deprofessionalising. *Nursing Times, 74,* 50–51.
5. Nurse, G. (1980) Counselling and helping skills: how can they be learned? *Nursing Times*, 24 April, 737–738.
6. Nurse, G. (1980b) *Counselling and The Nurse*, 2nd edn., Chap. 6, p.70. Aylesbury: H.M. & M.
7. Scammell, B.E. (1981) Communication? I've heard it all before. *Nursing, 27,* July, 1159–1161.
8. Givan, P. (1977) Healing and creative skills in counselling. *Nursing Times*, 18 August, 12–19.
9. Tschudin, V. (1982) *Counselling Skills for Nurses*, Chap. 3. p.31. London: Baillière Tindall.
10. Stewart, W. (1983) *Counselling in Nursing: A Problem Solving Approach*, Chap. 1, p.17. New York: Harper & Row.
11. Shipes, E.A. & Lehr, S.T. (1980) *Sexual Counselling for Ostomates*, Chap. 6, pp. 56–76. Springfield, Ill.: Charles C. Thomas.
12. Selby, J. (1985) Close encounters. *Nursing Times*, 8 May, 31.
13. Glover, J. (1982) Psychosexual counselling. *Nursing, No. 35,* March 1510–1511.

7 The influence of age on patients' problems

Patients who undergo surgery involving the creation of a stoma encounter a variety of problems: physical, physiological, psychological, and social.[1] Age undoubtedly colours the picture somewhat. The patient who has a stoma created as child is spared the psychological trauma of coping with changes in a long-standing body image and adaptation of established habits, whereas the patient who has a stoma created in later years does not encounter the difficulties of approaching schooling and adolescence being different from his peers.

Some problems remain almost universal throughout the age ranges. The need for information about the surgery and explanations regarding living with a stoma are common to all patients. Most age groups fear the reaction of their family and friends and have reservations and doubts about disclosing the fact that they have a stoma and explaining the need for its existence. Most patients appreciate sensitive support when they first look at the stoma and need reassurance that it is not easily damaged. While these problems may be virtually universal it must be remembered that all patients are very much individuals with their own personal frames of reference, and therefore their care must be individually tailored and the possible solutions to their problems carefully sought.

It is often beneficial to introduce a patient to an established patient with a stoma who has undergone similar surgery. Careful selection and matching of such a person is imperative and the patient associations are always willing to help by recommending a trained visitor for this purpose.[2] The family may also benefit from such an introduction so wives can talk to wives, parents to parents, and so on. Discussions with a well-established, positive stoma patient with whom the new patient can identify will enable him to realize that he is not alone; others have experienced and overcome similar problems to those he now faces. To facilitate this identification the visitor should be of a similar age and social background to the patient.

The nurse must work towards building a trusting relationship with the patient and his family to enable her to provide support and to facilitate effective counselling and empathetic nursing care.

BABIES

Stomas in babies are usually temporary to relieve intestinal obstruction in conditions such as Hirschsprung's disease or congenital anorectal abnormalities, as discussed in Chapters 2 and 3. There are far fewer babies than adults with stomas. Interestingly enough, however, it is believed that the first recorded successful colostomy was performed on a four-day old infant with anorectal agenesis by Duret in 1798.[3]

It is estimated that 250–300 infants have colostomies created annually in Britain.[4] The parents of these infants will be in need of explanation, psychological support, and counselling as they are the ones who will suffer the psychological problems associated with stomas, rather than the babies who are oblivious to the fact that they are 'different'. In many cases the stoma is closed before the child starts school.

Possible problems

Most parents will have limited knowledge about the nature and outcome of stoma surgery. They are the ones who will express anxiety on behalf of their offspring.[4] In a neonate the stoma is usually created as an emergency procedure, thus leaving little time for preoperative psychological preparation for his parents. The baby's mother is in the puerperal period and may already be feeling at a psychologically low ebb. If she had undergone a lengthy or difficult labour or has had a caesarean section she will be compromised physically and emotionally. Both parents will often be anxious about the hazards of surgery on a small baby and will be concerned about the risk to the infant's life.

The surgery may result in the mother and baby being separated at an early stage in the baby's life and this may interrupt maternal/infant bonding. The baby's parents will naturally be disappointed that their child is less than perfect and 'different' from their friends' offspring. They may experience feelings of guilt (particularly the mother). 'Was it something I did/did not do during my pregnancy?' is a common question. Some parents may have difficulty in accepting and relating to the baby who has an abnormality, particularly the father who does not have the benefit of maternal instincts.

The baby's grandparents, siblings, other family members and friends may also feel and possibly express emotions such as shock, disappointment, or morbid curiosity. If the child is to be offered for adoption it may be that he is more difficult to place.

Baby's skin is very sensitive and may become excoriated easily due to faecal contact. Selecting and fitting a suitable leak-proof appliance on a tiny but lively infant may pose a problem. Babies with a stoma, particularly those with an ileostomy, can become very quickly dehydrated if they suffer a gastrointestinal upset resulting in diarrhoea.[5] Anaemia can result from stoma bleeding particularly if the dietary intake of iron is low.

Specific nursing care

The parents should be given a full explanation of the condition and proposed treatment, with a description of the stoma and the possible implications. Ideally, this information should be presented to the parents preoperatively or, if this is not practical, at as early a stage as possible. An outline of the future planned care and support should also be given since frequent regular hospital visits may be involved. The fact that the stoma is temporary should also be emphasized. A booklet 'A Very Special Baby' is soon to be published by the Royal College of Nursing, compiled by members of a stoma care nursing course at Salford Hospital. It deals with many questions asked by parents of babies who have a stoma.

Sensitive counselling is essential and the parents should be encouraged to discuss and explore their feelings and share them with each other. The mother should be encouraged to handle and care for her baby as soon as possible after surgery. Teaching the parents to care for the stoma and surrounding skin at an early stage is also helpful. The baby's father should also be included in care as much as possible. Nurses should endeavour to express their acceptance of the baby with a stoma, not necessarily in words but by actions, facial expressions, and emotions. The parents should be encouraged to hold the baby close to them and give him the love and security he needs. Other family members may benefit from being involved in the care of the baby and may also need counselling, teaching, and explanation as appropriate.

The baby's skin must be meticulously cared for and protected at all times. In some areas the skin is cleaned and dried and then protected by an accurately cut barrier wafer. The mucosa of the stoma is covered with Vaseline gauze and an absorbent pad applied to collect effluent. This is held in place with a binder. However, with this method there is a risk of skin excoriation and trauma to the stoma due to friction.[4] It is preferable to fit a drainable appliance to collect the faeces and it is quite possible to fit a secure leakproof appliance to even the smallest baby.[4] The criteria is not the size of the appliance itself (which can be folded) but the type and area of adhesion. (See Chapters 4 and 17.)

Hospital attention may be required if an infant with a stoma (particularly an ileostomy) develops diarrhoea. The parents should be warned of what symptoms may occur and given clear instructions of what action to take in this situation. Regular haemoglobin checks should be made, particularly if the parents report stoma bleeding and the appropriate treatment, e.g. iron supplements given if indicated.

CHILDREN

Stomas may be created in children for a variety of conditions, they may be temporary or permanent, elective or emergency. See Chapters 2 and 3. The care planned for the child will vary depending upon the type of stoma and the child's predisposing condition. Both child (depending upon age) and parents will be in need of education and psychological support.

Possible problems

If the child has never been in hospital before he may be terrified of the unknown and have little idea of what is going to happen to him. The child and his parents will be unsure of both what surgery involves and what to expect regarding life with a stoma. All three will be anxious and fearful, needing time to accept the situation and absorb information; this time may be unavailable if the surgery is being carried out as an emergency. If the child is young or handicapped his parents may resent the nursing staff assuming responsibility for his physical care and feel excluded.

Early education is the foundation for future learning and if the child is ill he may miss long periods of school resulting in an interruption of this formative time. On return to school he may be unnecessarily excluded from activities such as sports and swimming by his teachers because he has a stoma. If the stoma was created in babyhood the child may be unaware he is 'different' until he attends school and mixes with other children. However, the older child may be acutely aware of his altered bodily function[6] and if his peers do not accept him into their group or tease him, he may develop psychological problems and become withdrawn or reluctant to go to school.

The child's parents may feel there is a social stigma as their child is different from his playmates. If the stoma is permanent and created electively they may also be worried that he will disagree with their decision regarding surgery when he is an adult. Children are naturally inquisitive and may ask questions which the parents feel incapable of answering adequately.

The child may fiddle with his appliance, and this may be a phase of natural development and exploration of his body or in the older child it may be a ruse, since the resulting leakage may provide him with an ideal excuse to avoid an unpopular task, such as a lesson he dislikes! Parents may treat their child as frail or as an invalid and attempt to restrict unduly his activities or allow his misbehaviour to continue unchecked. This can result in brothers and sisters resenting the special attention. In other families siblings may also encounter problems if their friends pass unkind comments or tease them about their brother or sister being different. This may result in a conflict between their instinct to go to the defence of their brother or sister and their anger that he is the cause of this unwanted attention being directed at them. Older family members may have difficulty in relating to the child as they are unsure how to react.

In some cases the child will develop unreasonable food fads using the stoma as an excuse to get his own way and avoid eating the food he dislikes, resulting in extra work for his mother and possible resentment from his brothers and sisters.

Specific nursing care

The child's parents should be encouraged to prepare him prior to hospital admission so that he is aware of what happens in hospital; the idea that it is an adventure should be promoted. Full explanation of surgery and treatment should be given to the parents and other family members if indicated. A plan of the help and support available should also be given. The child himself must be given an explanation in simple terms which his age level will allow him to understand, and this explanation may also be extended to his brothers and sisters.

Colouring books especially designed to help children to understand and accept a stoma are available and provide excellent material for the parents and nurses to assist the child to learn through play.[7] It is often helpful for smaller children to play with an appliance, putting it on a doll or teddy-bear to become familiar with a bag.[8] Again parents and nurses should be involved in these games and make it an opportunity to teach.

The child's parents should be encouraged to participate in his care as much as possible; if the mother is able to be resident at the hospital this is ideal. The child and his parents should be taught the care of the stoma and surrounding skin as soon as possible. Depending upon the age of the child he may be taught to carry out his own care independently, with his parents acting as supervisors. Even small children can participate in their own care, 'helping mum' by passing equipment and assisting in the procedure as much as they are able. This participation will help the child to learn to care for his stoma and often a five-year-old can learn to empty his own bag.

The teachers involved with the child may need explanation and education. The decision as to whether to accept the child in a school rests with the head teacher. Teaching staff involved with the child will require information about practical aspects of care as well as education about the child's physical abilities and limitations to avoid his activities being unduly restricted. The school can also be of help in liaising with teachers at the hospital to minimize the effect of time lost from school.

If the child has had the stoma from a young age he will have incorporated its existence into his body image during development. If peer group teasing is suspected the teacher may be able to help by observing the child's interactions with his peers. The teacher can then discourage any adverse reactions and alert parents if they feel other children are being cruel. Discussion with the parents of other children may also help in overcoming the problems of teasing.

Parents should be encouraged to discuss and share their feelings, fears and anxieties. The nurse should endeavour to build a trusting relationship with them and the child to enable her to provide maximum psychological support. 'Children have an enormous capacity for accepting their stoma. They must be treated honestly and respectfully.'[9] The child's parents should be encouraged to answer the child's questions in simple terms that he will understand, but they should always be truthful. Children will accept a simple explanation more readily than an evasive 'To make you better!'. The nurse may be able to prepare the parents by anticipating some of the possible questions and assisting the parents to formulate a suitable reply in advance.

Although the child should be allowed to handle and play with appliances and should participate in his stoma care he should be discouraged from interfering with his bag at other times. If leakage occurs this should be dealt with in a matter-of-fact manner with minimal fuss. The child may be testing the response to leakage or seeking attention. If it is suspected that the leaks are an excuse to avoid something particular a change should be executed as quickly as possible and the child then should attend the lesson or do the task so that his excuse proves unsuccessful.

The child's parents should be encouraged to treat the child as normally as possible. The parents should be taught that the child needs to play normally or be corrected if his behaviour is socially unacceptable.[5] If the mother is reluctant to allow the child to be treated normally this may be a sign of her own psychological need to have a dependent offspring. The other family members and siblings should also be encouraged to treat the child normally, which may help minimize resentment from brothers and sisters.[5] Older family members may also need education and support to equip them to relate to the child. Reading a pamphlet giving information about children with stomas may help here.[10]

Dietary restrictions for the child with a stoma should be minimal, as with all such patients. (See Chapter 16.) Parents should be advised to ignore food fads that bear no relation to any professional advice they have received and should encourage the child to eat a varied, balanced diet along with the rest of the family; this again promotes a sense of normality.

TEENAGERS

Stomas may be created in the teens for several conditions as discussed in Chapters 2 and 3. The teenager will be in need of a great deal of psychological support since the adolescent years are a period of change and adaptation and the creation of a stoma at this time can be particularly traumatic. Both the teenager and his parents will require explanation and support.

Possible problems

Puberty is a time when adaptation to an altered body image is already taking place. If there is also a stoma to be incorporated into this revised image then greater adaptation is required and will put extra pressures onto teenagers during this difficult time. During the teenage years there is an acute awareness of appearance, thus it can be very traumatic for a teenager to be 'different' from his peers. This may manifest as acute embarrassment after games lessons when communal showers pose a seemingly insurmountable problem, or it may be an anxiety about the ability to wear the latest fashion trend in clothes. No teenager will want to dress in loose clothes if all his friends are in sleek, fitted styles.

Schooling comes to its culmination during this time and exams are taken which often form the basis of a future career. An interruption in education may be a critical factor in the teenager's ultimate academic achievements. Parents and teenagers may have totally different anxieties regarding the stoma, for example parents are often more concerned with long-term problems, e.g. career, marriage, and parenthood, while the teenager is far more concerned with today and tomorrow, e.g. 'Can I play football?' 'Will the appliance show under my jeans?'.

The generation gap can often cause a communication barrier between a teenager and his parents, and this can cause a difficulty in discussion about the stoma or any other problem the teenager has, or his parents think he may have! The teenager may also see the nurse as a parent/teacher figure and thus assume that she will not understand. This may make him reluctant to talk openly about his feelings and anxieties and share them with her.

Teenagers not only need to identify with their peers in appearance, they also have a need for social acceptance, to feel part of the group. Teenagers worry about the reactions of their friends and, indeed, what they should tell people. 'How can I explain I have an ileostomy?' Once the teenager wishes to become involved in relationships with the opposite sex another set of problems arise. The teenager naturally wants to be seen as physically attractive and desirable; will this still be possible with a stoma? When to tell a prospective partner and what to say are also common anxieties. Most people beginning a physical relationship for the first time are very self-conscious and unsure, trying desperately to create the right impression yet unclear as to what is expected of them. The teenager with a stoma is more acutely aware of this uncertainty in their desire to be loved.

Specific nursing care

The teenager should be seen as an individual and given all the information he needs regarding his condition and surgery. He will need sensitive counselling sessions to enable him to express his feelings. Invariably teenagers will respond more readily if they are treated as adults as much as possible. The nurse should, however, be prepared for outbursts of childlike behaviour or 'psychological testing' ('How far can I go?'). These outbursts should be dealt with firmly as they arise, but should not prevent the teenager still being treated as an adult.

The teenager's parents will also need explanation and support. If the teenager is under 16 years they will need to give parental consent for the surgery. Discussion sessions as a family group are often productive as well as separate interviews. They can encourage openness and alleviate the suspicion of secrecy— teenagers are often distrustful of adults discussing them out of earshot. However, separate meetings with parents also provide an opportunity for them to share their feelings and be given any support they may need in dealing with problems. The nurse should endeavour to encourage open discussion rather than deception or subterfuge of any kind. The family may need this support and encouragement to enable them to break down any communication barriers.

The teachers at school can also be of help in overcoming problems regarding education. If there is a particular teacher the teenager relates to or a personal tutor, then liaison with him may be beneficial with regard to the patient returning to school and rehabilitation.

Teenagers are often very self-conscious about their body and appear to be secretive when changing the appliance or dealing with their stoma. This will need sensitive understanding by the nurse who should safeguard their privacy as much as possible. The teenager should be encouraged to experiment with clothes and appliances to enable him to be sure his bag is discreet and not detectable when wearing sleek styles. Information and tips on overcoming problems with clothing should be given. (See Chapter 17.)

The nurse must build up a relationship based on honesty and trust to facilitate frank discussion. The teenager should be encouraged to talk about his fears and reservations. He will need to talk about telling his friends and what he should say. It is sometimes helpful for the teenager to practice a short explanation on the nurse in an informal type of role-play to enable him to become familiar with the explanation and how he feels saying the words. This may allow him to have more confidence and thus appear more casual when he broaches the subject with his friends.

Extreme sensitivity is paramount when counselling the teenager regarding problems with physical relationships. He must be encouraged to talk about anticipated difficulties and work through them, seeking a possible solution that will work for him. He should be reminded that everyone is unsure initially in relationships and often his partner will be just as anxious as he is to create a good impression. The teenager should also be reminded that most people have several prospective partners before they find 'Mr Right'. It may not be the fact of the stoma that caused a relationship to flounder; don't his friends have romantic problems too? The question of when to tell is a very difficult one. Obviously it is not information he will want to impart during a first dance! However, if he waits until he is emotionally involved with a partner rejection can be more hurtful. If rejection does occur, this will make him even more reluctant to risk such a situation

happening again. There is no solution! The teenager has to learn
to judge when the time is right. Role-play again may help in
discovering what is best to say. A simple initial explanation is often
adequate with more detailed information being given as appropriate. It is usually accepted that it is far better for a prospective
partner to be told about a stoma before discovery is imminent.
Discovery of a stoma appliance is not associated only with sexual
intercourse and today with greater sexual freedom this problem is
quite relevant to teenage patients. Information and advice with
regard to contraception should also be made available if required.
(See Chapter 16.)

Teenage patients may also benefit from reading and discussing
pamphlets available from the United Ostomy Association on
sexual relationships.[11]

YOUNG ADULTS

Stomas in young adults are most commonly due to inflammatory
bowel disease and, therefore, tend to be ileostomies. However,
other causes are sometimes seen. (See Chapters 2 and 3.) The
problems faced by the young adult when having a stoma will, in
some cases, overlap those of the teenager and those in later life.

Specific problems

During one's twenties and thirties one may be completing
post-basic education and establishing a career. Time away through
illness may disrupt career plans and delay possible progress. The
patient may well be anxious about his job security if he is away
from work for long periods of time. A young wife and mother can
be very worried about her ability to cope with her children and run
a home after surgery.

The young adult will probably be unsure about what activities
will still be possible when he has a stoma. This can evoke doubts
about his social activities and recreational pastimes. Concern may
be expressed about the reaction of his friends and workmates to
his surgery and he could also experience doubts about explanations. He may be worried that the stoma will count against him if
he applies for a job or seeks promotion; should he disclose the fact
that he has a stoma to prospective employers?

One of the most severe anxieties the patient has is often concern
about the partner's response. Those with a steady relationship fear

rejection from their loved one, while others worry about forming lasting relationships. Worries about sexual problems both physical and psychological are also common, as are fears regarding fertility, pregnancy, and parenthood. A frequent question is 'Is my condition hereditary?'. If the patient is already a parent he may worry about the reaction of his young children, how to explain the stoma and satisfy their childlike curiosity.

Specific nursing care

The patient will require detailed information of his proposed surgery and should be informed about the possibility of living a full and rewarding life with a stoma. He will still be able to go out for a beer with the boys or enjoy a special meal at a restaurant, go to parties, and play sport. It is often helpful if the partner can be included in these discussions. However, the patient should also be given the opportunity to express his feelings in confidence. Clear instruction about what activities should be avoided and for how long after surgery must be given. The patient should also be reassured that almost all activities are still possible after having a stoma following a suitable period of convalescence.

Early assessment of the home or employment circumstances will help the nurse to plan the patient's rehabilitation and organize support if it is needed, e.g. day nursery attendance for children. Is there an occupational health nurse at the place of employment who may be able to assist the patient when he returns to work, e.g. providing facilities for an emergency appliance change? Naturally, nobody outside the medical and nursing teams should be approached without the patient's explicit permission. Counselling regarding explaining his condition (who to tell, when and how) should take place to prepare the patient for the questions he will undoubtedly face. If the patient is unsure regarding the reaction of a young family and feels uncertain of how to answer their questions this will need exploration and, possibly, rehearsal. The patient should be reminded that young children are resilient and will accept simple, honest explanations. With regard to employment the patient should be advised to disclose the fact that he has a stoma if he is asked at an employment medical. He should, however, emphasize that he has been effectively cured of any disease by removal of the organ if appropriate, for instance patients who have had ulcerative colitis and have undergone panproctocolectomy can be said to be cured.

Patients should be encouraged to talk about their feelings and anxieties. The nurse should encourage the patient to discuss his feelings with his partner and explain his reservations. The partner should be encouraged to look at the stoma, having previously been warned that the patient will be watching intently for any sign of revulsion either by word or gesture. It may prove helpful if the nurse stays with the couple at this time to lend moral support. By offering sensitive, diplomatic support and encouraging frank discussion the nurse can often help to avert a lot of anxieties on behalf of both partners. Some simple, practical suggestions regarding their physical relationship (if appropriate) may also be helpful, as can reassurance regarding fertility, contraception, and pregnancy. (See Chapter 16.)

The aim should be to enable the patient to realize that they are a normal wife/mother or husband/father who happens to have a stoma.[12] The stoma must be accommodated into their lifestyle, rather than them make a brave attempt to fit an altered and possibly resented lifestyle around the stoma.

MIDDLE AGE

The middle-aged patient may have an ileostomy, colostomy, or urinary stoma; in this age group a whole variety of diseases resulting in ostomy surgery can occur. (See Chapters 2 and 3.) Life is said to begin at 40, as often families are growing, careers are established, a regular domestic pattern has evolved alongside a stable long-standing partnership. This creates a scenario of security and a settled lifestyle. Middle age is a time of change beginning with growing families leaving the nest, physical changes in appearance, menopause, the acceptance of growing older and preparing for retirement. All these factors can put pressure onto the patient to adapt his lifestyle.

If a stoma is created at this time when these other adjustments may already be under way, further adaptation is required leading the patient to view the future from a different prospective, seeking recognition that they are still the same person.[13]

Possible problems

The patient will probably be unsure of what adjustments he may have to make to his lifestyle when he has a stoma and this can pose a threat to his psychological security. He will be unsure of what activities having a stoma will curtail. If this is coupled with the other adaptations being made in middle age further resentment towards having a stoma can result in adverse psychological effects. The patient may also blame the stoma for his having to curtail certain activities or generally slow down due to the natural ageing process.

The patient with an established career may well be concerned about missing time at work. Will they manage without me? Will somebody younger step into my place? Will I be able to resume my previous role after surgery? Will they put me out to grass in a menial position or pension me off? Will I be made redundant? These are all common fears the patient may voice. Employment doubts can lead to a great deal of anxiety particularly if the patient is the sole breadwinner with financial commitments. He may see this as a further threat to his established lifestyle. Female patients may equally worry about the family coping without them: who will cook the meals, wash the clothes, clean, and remember to pay the bills? Everybody has a need for recognition and status. We all like to feel we are indispensable and the reality that life can go on without us being available can come as quite a shock. This can be a severe blow to the patient's ego. Other worries about dependants, possibly elderly parents, can also impair the patient's own well-being.

The middle-aged patient also faces fears of rejection by the partner and can see the stoma as a threat to his relationship. Sexual problems may result from physical causes such as impotence due to parasympathetic nerve damage[14] or dyspareunia due to altered vaginal anatomy or scar tissue.[15] Other problems are due to psychological factors such as poor self-esteem or fear of damaging the stoma. Sexual function in middle age may be waning naturally but the stoma may be put forward as the cause or attributed with the blame. (See Chapter 16.)

The patient will often express worries about the reaction of his family, friends and colleagues. A particular worry may be about the response of teenage offspring who are often very sensitive and do not like their parents to be in any way different from the parents of their friends. There may already be communication difficulties in a growing family and the patient may be at a loss as to how to explain and handle this situation. If he faces an adverse reaction from his offspring this may compound his fears of confiding in those outside his immediate family circle.

Specific care

The patient, his partner, and often his children will all need explanation, counselling, reassurance and support. The patient may well need to explore his own feelings about his present lifestyle, the possible changes the future will bring and how he will cope with these adaptations. He will often need help in accepting that the stoma is not a barrier to the continuation of his life where he left off before surgery. Discussion with the patient about possible employment worries, financial difficulties and domestic problems may encourage him to evaluate his fears. Sensitive counselling can enable the patient to explore his feelings and ascertain what his actual problems are; he can then be helped to consider the possible alternative solutions.

As the patient may be feeling insecure because he has a stoma, which he sees as a threat to his lifestyle, he will need diplomatic support to enable him to retain his need for status and leave his ego unscathed. The family should also be cautioned about this need and warned that the patient may be particularly sensitive. If there are practical problems with financial or domestic arrangements then the patient can be helped by an experienced social worker who can arrange to obtain the appropriate help. The suggestion of seeing a social worker must be made tactfully as some patients may be sensitive and associate this with a social stigma. Counselling regarding family problems and communication could be indicated and the patient may use the nurse as a sounding board to test out his explanations and ideas.

Great sensitivity and empathy are needed to enable the patient to realize that his established lifestyle will need to change and adapt as he grows older and that it may not often be the fact he has a stoma that is the cause of this change.

THE ELDERLY

The elderly patient is most likely to have a colostomy, which may be permanent or temporary depending upon the predisposing condition. (See Chapters 2 and 3.) Many of the problems encountered by younger patients still have to be faced but these may be compounded by diminished physical ability and declining mental agility. The elderly patient with a stoma often fears change and experiences difficulty in adapting to alterations in the habits of a lifetime.

Possible problems

The elderly often relate to experiences in the past, thus his knowledge of surgery, anaesthesia, and living with a stoma is often outdated but none the less deeply ingrained into his memory.[16] He may have known somebody years ago who underwent surgery resulting in a stoma and experienced severe problems resulting in a very poor quality of life. In later life the fear of death is often more imminent and the elderly patient worries whether he will survive major surgery or, indeed, he wonders if it is worth while; would he be better to die?

The body image develops in early life and the longer the patient has held this image the more difficult it is to incorporate change. The patient has often followed a routine of personal hygiene and bowel habit for many years; how can he alter this now? It is not so many years ago that subjects such as bowel function and, more particularly, sex were taboo, thus the patient feels that he cannot talk freely about such things, particularly to a nurse he sees as being young enough to be his grandchild. Sexual activity is important for emotional and general well-being. However, attitudes often inhibit sexual activity in the elderly and myths that sexual interest wanes in later middle age and stops after retirement, for instance, are widely believed. Society in general, the elderly themselves, and professional carers may believe sexual intercourse in old age to be harmful to health, unnatural, and 'not nice'.[17] The patient may wish to maintain his modesty, thus he feels he cannot disclose his feelings. The elderly patient may find it hard to make the effort to chat and socialize; he can quickly become isolated and lonely.[18]

Some elderly people cling to their independence and fear that a stoma will result in their being no longer able to care for themselves in their own homes. Conversely others may use the stoma as an excuse to become dependent and cared for in their old age. The patient may well fear for the well-being of his elderly partner while he is in hospital. It may be that the spouse is not in good health and cannot cope alone. The capacity to learn wanes with age and it may take the elderly patient a long time to learn the care of his stoma and to change his appliance. Failing eyesight, lack of dexterity, or decreased mental ability may make it impossible for the patient to undertake his own care thus threatening his independence.

Bowel function in the elderly may be sluggish, as long as eight days can elapse from ingestion of food to defecation in the elderly hospital patient.[19] Coupled with this can often be a minimal fluid intake, i.e. 1–2 pints daily.[20] The elderly patient with a colostomy is, therefore, as prone to constipation as any other elderly patient but the prevention and treatment of the constipation requires careful planning.

Specific care

It is important to elicit whether the patient has any previous knowledge or preconceived ideas regarding the planned surgery. If these are positive they can be reinforced and used as a basis for teaching. However, if the ideas are negative or outdated then the nurse should work towards dispelling them and educating the patient. The patient should be reassured about the safety of modern surgery and anaesthesia, although false promises must never be made. He should be encouraged to talk about his fears. The elderly patient will require more time to absorb the information that he needs, and he may require facts repeating several times. The nurse must respect the patient's age and avoid talking down to him and giving reassurance as if he were a child.

Sensitive support and counselling will be needed to enable the elderly patient to accept the alteration in his body's image and to adapt gradually to new habits. The nurse must be particularly diplomatic when broaching subjects such as bowel function and sex which the patient may have difficulty discussing openly. It will take time for the nurse to establish a trusting relationship in which the elderly patient feels comfortable to confide, without feeling embarrassed.

The patient's independence must be preserved whenever possible and every effort should be made to enable him to retain his self-respect by learning to care for his own stoma. Tendencies towards becoming dependent upon the nursing staff should be discouraged; the nurse must be firm and positive about his retaining independence.

The elderly patient should be taught an uncomplicated stoma care routine as soon as possible.[16] It is essential that an appliance is chosen that is easy for the patient to prepare and apply. (See Chapter 4.) The elderly patient will need time and encouragement when learning to care for his stoma and the nurse must consider his physical and mental limitations. In some cases the patient may not be able to carry out his own stoma care either because of senility or physical incapacitation. In this case a relative may be taught to undertake the care, or it will be carried out by nursing staff after discharge.

If the patient is anxious about the welfare of his elderly partner it may be possible to arrange social support or short-term care until he is well enough to cope again. Voluntary helpers who will visit, shop, or provide transport may also prove valuable to the elderly couple. Information about the patient's domestic circumstances is also vital to the nurse to enable her to plan care after discharge and rehabilitation. Social Services may need to arrange home help, meals on wheels and other support if required.

REFERENCES

1. Devlin, H.B., Plant, J.A., & Griffin, M. (1971) The aftermath of surgery for ano-rectal cancer. *British Medical Journal, iii*, 413.
2. Colostomy Welfare Group, 39 Eccleston Square (2nd Floor), London SW1V IPB; Ileostomy Association, Central Office, Amblehurst House, Chobham, Woking, Surrey GU24 8PZ; Urostomy Association, c/o Mrs V. Kings, 8 Coniston Close, Dane Bank, Denton, Manchester, M34 2EW.
3. Richardson, R.G. (1973) *The Abominable Stoma*. Chap. 2, pp.3–4. Abbott Laboratories Ltd.
4. Lister, J., Webster, P.J., & Mirza, S. (1983) Colostomy complications in children. *The Practitioner* February, *227*, 229–237.
5. Nethercott, S.G. & Williams, D.J. (1982) Parents as nurses. In *Community View*. September *17*. Smith & Nephew Ltd.
6. McNemar, A. (1972) A child's incorporation of changes in body image following ileal loop diversion. *Maternal–Child Nursing Journal, 1*, 33–38.
7. Kirkland, S. (1985) Ostomy dolls for paediatric patients. *Journal of Enterostomal Therapy, 12*, No. 3, 104–105.
8. Webster, P. (1985) Special babies. *Community Outlook*, July. 19–22.
9. Held, D., & Klostermann, A. (1983) *Chris has an Ostomy*. International Ostomy Association.
10. '*My Child Has An Ostomy*' International Ostomy Association.
11. Binder, D.P. (1973) *Sex, Courtship and the Single Ostomate*. International Ostomy Association.

12. Brewster, L. (1984) Keeping in touch. *Nursing Mirror*, 9 December, *159*, 8–9.
13. Bourke, R. (1984) Thriving with a stoma. *Nursing Mirror*, 9 December, *159*, 5–6.
14. Devlin, H.B. & Plant, J. (1979) Sexual function—an aspect of stoma care part II. *British Journal of Sexual Medicine*. March, 22–25.
15. Brouillette, N.J., Pryor, E. & Fox, T.A.Jr. (1981) Evaluation of sexual dysfunction in the female following rectal resection and intestinal stoma. In *Disease of the Colon and Rectum*, Chap 24, pp.96–102.
16. Model, G. (1984) Focus on the elderly. *Nursing Mirror* 9 December *159*, No. 9, 2–4.
17. Wright D. (1985) Sex and the Elderly. *Nursing Mirror*, 31 July *161*, No. 5, 18–19.
18. Model, G. (1983) Focus on the elderly stoma patient. *Proceedings of Nursing Mirror/RCN Society of Geriatric Nursing International Conference.* Squibb Surgicare Ltd. September.
19. Brocklehurst, J.C., et al. (1969) A study of faecal stasis in old age and the use of dorbanex. *Gerontology Clinics, 11*, 293–300.
20. Anderson, J. (1984) Bowel function in the elderly. *Nursing Times*, August, 52.

8 Preoperative stoma care

The patient who is to undergo surgery that involves the creation of a stoma faces many problems. Many of his anxieties are born of uncertainty and lack of knowledge. The preoperative care that is planned for the patient will not only depend upon him as an individual but also upon the predisposing disease and the circumstances prior to surgery. A patient who has had a long history of ulcerative colitis which has resulted in long-standing ill health and a poor quality of life, may well view the prospect of having a stoma as a very small price to pay for good health and the ability to lead an active life again. Conversely, the patient who noticed spots of blood when he passed a motion may have visited his family doctor suspecting he had haemorrhoids; the fact that he is now told by a surgeon he needs a major operation to remove his back passage and leave a colostomy may be incomprehensible.

If the surgery is to be undertaken as a planned procedure this will allow adequate time for psychological as well as physical preparation. However, when the surgery is to be performed in an emergency situation little if any time is available for explanations and reassurance, in addition the patient is usually very ill and may well be in pain. The patient who has the benefit of preoperative explanation and counselling and the opportunity to ask questions and discuss his feelings will often accept his stoma more readily after surgery and be rehabilitated more quickly than a patient who has not had the benefit of adequate psychological preparation.[1] The patient undergoing stoma surgery has numerous adjustments to make. How well he makes those adjustments depends a great deal on the nursing care he receives in the hospital.[2]

When formulating a plan of care for the patient the nurse must take into consideration what possible problems and anxieties he faces. He may not have even heard of a stoma, let alone be aware of what one is and the implications this may have on his lifestyle. What does it look like? How big is it? Where on my body will it be? Will it show? These are all common questions asked by patients in need of explanation. The response of one patient told she needed surgery was: 'A colostomy! I didn't like the sound of that, though I wasn't really sure what it was.'[3]

The patient may not have retained all the information given to him by the doctor because he was too shocked, frightened, or overawed to absorb facts. He may be unaware of what exactly the surgery involves and why it is necessary. The patient may be fearful of coming into hospital; he may have family, social, or financial problems which he feels will be compounded by a hospital admission. He may have no idea of how long he will be in the hospital. Fear of the unknown can manifest itself in a variety of psychological responses and the patient may feel ill at ease, threatened, or insecure. (See Chapter 5.) Often he will have many doubts and questions regarding life with a stoma that he may feel unable to verbalize. Doubts about bodily function, work, hobbies, social activities, and the reaction of others may be appearing as insurmountable obstacles to be faced.

Previous knowledge regarding life with a stoma may be a mixed blessing. If the patient knows somebody who has undergone similar surgery and now leads a full and active life, this may be very reassuring but if the knowledge the patient has is outdated or is of a person who suffered many complications and has not adjusted to having a stoma this may be counterproductive. It may be that the patient has never met anyone else who has a stoma. The idea of wearing a 'bag' can conjure up a variety of horrific images to an anxious patient who has no conception of what a modern stoma-care appliance looks and feels like. Again, outdated knowledge can further alarm the patient if he imagines he will be wearing a bulky appliance of yesteryear with no odour barrier at all.

Information about postoperative care and procedures is also important if the patient is to go for his operation fully aware of what to expect afterwards. It can be very alarming for the patient and his visiting family if he awakens to find himself attached to various tubes or machines he had no warning about. The patient's family will also naturally be apprehensive about his treatment and aftercare.

The patient is often subjected to rigorous bowel preparations which he may find uncomfortable and exhausting. To ensure the bowel is clean prior to surgery it is commonly necessary to severely restrict the dietary intake, in particular those foods high in residue.

PREOPERATIVE NURSING AIMS AND OBJECTIVES

1. Establish a comfortable rapport between nurse and patient to provide an open channel for communication and counselling.
2. Explain the service of care and support that is available so that the patient is aware of what help is available to him.
3. Provide opportunities for counselling to enable the patient to explore his problems and seek a solution.
4. Explain the surgery and care fully to the patient so he is wholly aware of what is going to happen to him.
5. Introduce patient to ward environment and other patients to enable him to feel at ease in the unfamiliar surroundings.
6. Involve the patient's family in his care and ensure that they have the information and support they require.
7. Supply the patient with suitable reading material about adapting to life with a stoma and other pertinent information.
8. Assess the patient's attitude towards the surgery and his feelings about having a stoma.
9. Introduce the patient to a suitable visitor who has undergone similar surgery.
10. Demonstrate and discuss appliances and assess the patient's particular needs. Fit an appliance to help establish a suitable stoma site.
11. Explain the need for thorough bowel preparation and dietary restrictions.
12. Explain fully the postoperative procedures so that the patient is fully conversant with what to expect after his operation.

Ideally the specialist nurse should make contact with the patient as soon as possible after the surgeon has told him that he will need surgery involving a stoma. In many cases this occurs in the outpatient department. The patient is often shocked at the news and capable of absorbing little information, therefore lengthy explanations are inappropriate. The aim of this initial interview is one of introduction. The stoma care support that is available should be outlined to the patient and any urgent questions may be answered. A further meeting should then be arranged, which may take place at the patient's home if the stoma care nurse visits in the community. A preoperative home visit allows the patient to talk to the nurse on his own territory where he is more likely to feel relaxed.[1] It also provides the nurse with an opportunity to ascertain the patient's home circumstances and facilities. An opportunity to assess the family relationships and interactions is also valuable and the nurse may be able to meet other family members. The nurse can then make a nursing assessment and begin to plan the patient's care.

Once a comfortable rapport has been established, preoperative counselling can begin to allow the patient to explore and express his fears and anxieties. The nurse can gradually give the patient the information he needs to enable him to seek a satisfactory solution to his problems. If no nurse specialist is available the nurse in the outpatient department may be able to lessen the patient's anxiety by offering reassurance and outlining the expected plan of events. It is often helpful if the patient can be given the telephone number of a professional to contact in case he has any pressing questions or doubts. An introduction to the nursing staff on the ward to which he is to be admitted may also help to lessen anxiety.

A meeting with a patient who has undergone similar surgery is often very helpful in promoting positive attitudes. Careful matching of age, sex, social class, and lifestyle is most helpful in enabling the patient to identify with the visitor. There are various voluntary organizations set up by patients with stomas as self-help groups which will arrange for a trained visitor to contact the patient and talk to him both before and after his operation. (See Chapter 12.)

The patient may also like to read a booklet about his proposed surgery as this can act as a stimulus for further questions. However, the nurse must be aware that the patient can be overwhelmed if too much information is given too quickly and he may attempt to learn and retain all the information in the booklet, which can place an extra burden on his already strained mental state. It is important to make sure the patient realizes that the booklet is only another source of information and advice and should not be regarded as a strict rule book, nor should the nurse assume that this reading will provide all the information the patient needs thus making discussion unnecessary. Several manufacturers of stoma appliances produce these booklets which are often written with the help of experienced stoma care nurses.[4]

The stoma care nurse should endeavour to meet the patient as soon as possible after he is admitted. This can be very helpful in enabling the patient to settle in since there will be at least one nurse whom he recognizes and to whom he can relate. If there is no nurse specialist for stoma care patients, the ward nurse responsible for the patient's care should endeavour to put him at ease, show him around the ward and introduce him to fellow patients. The first few hours spent in hospital can be particularly stressful to the patient as he is in an alien environment amongst strangers.

Whilst getting to know the patient and putting him at ease, the nurse should be gathering the necessary information she requires to make a full nursing assessment. (See Appendix I at the end of this chapter.) This can be achieved in an informal manner; while the nurse is helping the patient to settle she can use her eyes, ears, nose and hands to gain an impression of the patient.[5] The collection of information must never take the form of an interrogation and the nurse must convey confidentiality.

During her contact with the patient the nurse should discuss the patient's attitude towards surgery and elicit whether he has any preconceived ideas about life with a stoma. Positive attitudes should be reinforced whilst outdated ideas should be discussed and the patient made aware of improvements. The nurse should find out what the patient understands about his proposed surgery and build onto the explanation given by the surgeon so that the patient is fully aware of what is to happen. Drawing a simple diagram to clarify the explanation is often very helpful. Information regarding postoperative procedures, tubes and drains should also be given.

The patient should be given a clear explanation of what a stoma is and how it works. He may also benefit from seeing pictures or slides of a stoma and other topics such as appliances and patients with stomas enjoying life's activities.[6] A suitable set of slides is available from a manufacturer of stoma appliances together with a explanatory catalogue.[7] These pictures should only be shown to the patient after a full explanation if he wishes it, otherwise he may find them somewhat alarming.

After sensitive preparation the patient should be shown the various types of appliance. After considering his needs, the nurse should help the patient to assess which appliance he feels he would like to wear. The patient should also be shown the type of appliance that will be fitted in the immediate postoperative period, that is a *drainable* bag made from *clear* plastic.

It is helpful when assessing a suitable position for the stoma if the patient wears an appliance containing 100 ml water to assess comfort.[7] Once a suitable site has been established it should be marked indelibly on the skin. (See Chapter 9.)

All the patient's questions should be answered simply and honestly. The nurse must, however, avoid giving false reassurance. If the patient is given too much information too quickly he will be unable to absorb and retain it. However, if the patient asks too many questions at once the nurse must be careful not to appear evasive. She should ensure he is aware that she will talk to him regularly and give him lots of opportunities to discuss his doubts. The nurse should also acknowledge hearing the questions and express her intention of giving an explanation at a future meeting. A response such as 'I'm glad you asked me about diet, it is an important point. I thought that we could discuss food more fully after your operation. However, is there a particular question about eating you wanted to ask?' is often successful in postponing a discussion until another time. If the patient asks a difficult question which the nurse is unsure how to answer, she should again tell the patient that she is willing to answer his question but first must gain further information for herself. 'What makes you think that?' is a possible response to allow the nurse to assess more about the patient's reason for asking.

The nurse should look for 'messages' from the patient by action, expression or gesture that there may be more to be discussed. She should then help the patient to express his feelings and anxieties and encourage open discussion.

The patient will need help in many ways. He will require much reassurance whilst undergoing the rigours of bowel preparation; the importance of thoroughly cleansing the bowel to reduce postoperative morbidity must be simply emphasized. Although the diet must be necessarily low in residue it should be made as appetizing as possible and several proprietary, nutritious, low residue, palatable preparations are readily available.

Good communication is very important to establish a relationship with the patient's family as well as the patient so that they can be supported.[8] The patient's family and friends will be in need of explanation and reassurance. They will need an opportunity to express their fears and anxieties. It may be helpful to the patient and his spouse if they are both present at some of the preoperative counselling sessions, as well as being given the opportunity for confidential discussion. Those people who are close to the patient can play an important role in influencing the patient's own attitudes, and family involvement is therefore essential. The patient going for operation after adequate preoperative preparation should be totally *au fait* with what he is to expect after surgery.

REFERENCES

1. Stewart, L. (1984) Stoma care: pre-operative preparation of the patient. *Nursing, 30*, 886–7.
2. Doering, K.J. & Mountain, P.L. (1984) Ostomy Patients Part 1: Pre-op. Assessment. *Nursing 84*, September, 47–49.
3. Dorr Mullen, B. & McGinn, K.A. (1980) *The Ostomy Book*, Chap. 1, p.2. Palo Alto: Bull Publishing Co.
4. Abbott Laboratories Ltd, Queenborough, Kent ME11 5EL; Coloplast Ltd, Bridge House, Orchard Lane, Huntingdon, Cambs PE18 6QT; Squibb Surgicare Ltd, Squibb House, 141–149 Staines Road, Hounslow TW3 3JA; Franklin Medical, High Wycombe, Bucks HP12 3BR; Eschmann Bros & Walsh Ltd, Peter Road, Lancing, West Sussex BN15 8TJ.
5. Long, R. (1980) *Systematic Nursing Care*, Chap. 2, p.30. London: Faber & Faber.
6. Wilson, E. & Desruisseaux, B. (1983) Stoma care and patient teaching. *Patient Teaching*, Chap. 6, pp. 95–118. Ed. Wilson Barnett, J. Churchill Livingstone.
7. Cambmac Instruments Ltd., Denny Industrial Estate, Denny End Road, Waterbeach, Cambridge C85 9PY.
8. Goligher, J.C. (1984) *Surgery of the Anus, Rectum & Colon*, 5th edn. Chap. 22, p.860. London: Baillière Tindall.
9. Snee, N. (1979) Families of cancer patients. *Journal of Human Nutrition, 3*, 388–391.

APPENDIX I

Information to be included in a comprehensive stoma care nursing history

Initially general information is required.

Name

- What does he/she like to be called?

Address

- Type of house, e.g. bungalow/flat/house?
- Facilities at home, e.g. bathroom/toilet—separate/outside? Running water?

- Services in area?
- Who else occupies home?

Date of birth

- Age?

This can then be followed by more detailed information about the patient's family situation.

Family situation

- Married? Divorced? Widowed?
- Living alone or with others?
- What family does patient have?
- What family support is available?
- Do family have regular contact?
- Are family aware of illness?
- What is family's reaction to illness?
- What family commitments has patient got?
- What are family relationships like?
- Has he/she discussed illness with his/her family?

Discussion about the patient's occupation and status should also help the nurse to ascertain if the patient has any worries about his job.

Occupation

- Is patient employed?
- What is patient's occupation?

If employed:

- Is this his/her usual type of job?
- What exactly does work entail?
- What is work environment like?
- What facilities are available at work?
- What are work relationships like?
- Is there an occupational health nurse?
- Are there any financial difficulties while off work?
- Is he/she worried about his/her job security whilst off work?

- Is he/she worried about maintaining job status whilst away?
- Is he/she worried about any other aspect of his/her work (e.g. how will the family manage?)
- Has he/she discussed illness with his/her employer?

If unemployed:

- What was previous employment?
- Is this the type of work he/she wants to pursue?
- Why did job cease, e.g. redundancy, sickness?
- How does he/she feel about being unemployed, e.g. bored, bitter, resentful, depressed or worthless?
- Is there financial hardship?
- Is he/she actively seeking work?
- Does he/she fill his/her day with other activities, if so, what?

If housewife:

- Is she worried about family coping?
- Is she worried about status?
- Is she worried about financial matters?
- Is she worried about coping when she goes home?

If retired:

- What type of work did he/she do?
- How long has he/she been retired?
- How does he/she feel about retirement?
- Does he/she fill his/her day with other activities, if so, what?

Talking to the patient about his social activities, interests and hobbies will help to put him at ease, as well as providing the nurse with a valuable insight into her patient's lifestyle.

Social information

- What are his/her hobbies/interests?
- What do these entail?
- Does he/she play any sports?
- What does this involve?
- Does he/she go out socially?
- What sort of places does he/she go to?

- What type of holiday does he/she go on?
- Does he/she like to drink alcohol?
- If so, how much? Is this beer?
- How often does he/she go out?
- Does he/she have regular visitors?
- Does he/she have a close circle of friends—many acquaintances—or both?
- Does he/she have a particularly close friend?

Some patients have very strong religious beliefs and gain great comfort from faith and prayer, whilst others place little or no emphasis on religious belief. The nurse should endeavour to find out if the patient is a religious person and, if so, what implications his faith will have for her proposed care?

Religion

- Does he/she practice his/her religion?
- Does he/she have a close relationship with clergy?
- Does his/her faith have implications upon his/her life with a stoma? e.g. Islamic praying/ritual cleansing.

When broaching the subject of personal relationships the nurse must be sensitive to the patient's reactions to her questions and must never give the impression of prying. This information is essential to enable the nurse to see the patient in a holistic manner and forms a basis for counselling the patient regarding potential sexual problems and anxieties.

Personal relationships

- Is he/she married or has he/she an intimate relationship?
- Is the relationship stable?
- Does the partner know about the illness?
- What is the partner's reaction to the illness? How does he/she usually react to illness?
- Is the patient worried about his/her intimate relationships?
- What are the usual sleeping arrangements?
- Does he/she feel a stoma will affect his/her intimate relationships?
- What method of contraception does he/she use?

- Does he/she have any previous sexual problems?
- Has he/she discussed feelings/illness with his/her partner?
- Is he/she worried about forming future relationships?
- Is he/she heterosexual?

The patient's activities relating to daily living and bodily function must also be considered. This will enable the nurse to consider any limitations when planning the patient's care.

Activities relating to daily living/physical attributes

- Can he/she manage all aspects of personal hygiene unaided?
- What is his/her standard of hygiene?
- What is his/her usual hygiene routine?
- Is he/she fully ambulant without aid?
- Is he/she capable of strenuous physical activity?
- What is his/her eyesight like?
- What is his/her hearing like?
- What is his/her manual dexterity like?
- Does he/she receive any regular help with daily activities?
- Does he/she need any further help?
- What is bowel function like—does he/she ever get diarrhoea or constipation? If so what does he/she take for this?
- Has there been a change in bowel function?
- What is urinary function like?
- Has there been a change in urinary function?
- What is sleep pattern like?
- Has there been any change in sleep pattern?
- Does he/she wear any prosthesis?

Information about the patient's usual eating habits will equip the nurse to modify any advice she gives regarding diet to fit in with the patient's previous eating pattern.

Diet

- What is his/her appetite like?
- What is his/her usual eating pattern?
- What foods does he/she like?
- What foods does he/she dislike?

- What foods does he/she usually eat?
- Do any foods upset his/her system?
- In what way?
- Are there any foods he/she avoids?
- Why? If there is a reaction, what happens?
- Is he/she on a special diet?

The nurse must be aware of which medical practitioners are responsible for the patient's treatment and what type of relationship the patient has with his doctor. Information about the patient's previous medical history is also essential as this may influence his planned care, as may any medications he is taking.

Medical information

- Who is the GP?
- Who is the surgeon?
- What is the diagnosis?
- What is the prognosis?
- What treatment is planned?
- What previous illnesses has he/she had?
- What was his/her reaction?
- Has he/she had previous surgery?
- What was his/her reaction?
- How well does he/she know his/her GP?
- How well does he/she know his/her surgeon?
- What services are available in the community?

Drugs

- What drugs is he/she taking—type and dose?
- Why is he/she taking them?
- Is he/she allergic to any drug, food, or substance that he/she knows of?

Discussion regarding the patient's preference in styles of clothing will help the nurse in siting the stoma and in assisting in the selection of a suitable appliance.

Clothing

- What type of clothes does he/she prefer?
- Does he/she wear a corset or support?
- Does he/she have any worries about styles of clothing he/she can wear?
- Where does he/she usually buy his/her clothes?

For the nurse to give support and information to the patient's family and friends she needs to be aware of what the patient's wishes and intentions are:

Information given to others

- Who has he/she told about his/her illness?
- What has he/she told them?
- Who does he/she plan to tell?
- Does he/she want anyone to talk to any of his/her friends/ relatives?
- Is there any information he/she does not want disclosing?

The nurse must make a comprehensive assessment of the patient's psychological reaction to having a stoma and also of his personality and demeanour. This will form a basis on which to plan psychological support and lead into the counselling.

Psychological implications

- What is his/her disposition, e.g. cheerful/withdrawn?
- What is his/her general attitude?
- Is he/she open or reserved?
- What does he/she understand about his/her illness?
- Does he/she need more information?
- Has he/she ever heard of a stoma before?
- Does he/she know anyone with a stoma? If so, when, how do they cope? Is this positive or negative knowledge?
- What are his/her thoughts about having a stoma?
- How does he/she feel?
- Has he/she talked to anyone about his/her feelings? If so who?
- What does he/she think causes his/her feelings?
- How does he/she think he/she will cope?

● What does he/she think may help?

Finally the nurse should make a physical assessment of the patient.

Physical assessment

● Weight.
● Physique.
● Posture.
● Dexterity.
● Skin type
● Hair/eye (colour).
● Disposition (psychological).
● Disposition (physical).
● Intelligence.
● General health.

Although this appears to be a lengthy list of questions, not all the information has to be collected at the same time. Much of this data can be obtained during purposeful conversation over several occasions. Once established, the information will give an invaluable profile of the patient as an individual. It will provide a basis on which changes after surgery can be assessed and will enable the nurse to consider the needs of the individual when planning his care.

9 Choosing the site for a stoma

The choice of position for an ileostomy, colostomy or urinary stoma is of critical importance. Ideally, the site at which the stoma will be raised should be predetermined by an experienced person after careful consideration.[1] Some surgeons will allow a trained stoma care nurse to mark the stoma site after due consultation with himself and discussion with the patient.[2] Other surgeons prefer to undertake this task personally, or come to a decision jointly with a trained nurse.

The patient's ability to lead a full and active life will be greatly compromised if the stoma is misplaced. To ensure that the patient can be confident and comfortable in the future with an appliance that does not leak and with healthy peristomal skin, an appliance should be fitted and the site 'tested' prior to surgery.[3] This decision can have such a profound effect on the patient's postoperative rehabilitation that it is of the utmost importance that the site chosen is suitable.

Experience has shown it is advisable to mark a prospective stoma site whenever there is a possibility of creating a stoma, for instance anterior resection where possible temporary defunctioning of the distal colon may be required (as already discussed in a previous chapter). The patient should be assured that the stoma, if created, will be temporary. Although this may be said to cause unnecessary anxiety at the time it can protect the patient from the effects of a misplaced stoma.

It may at times be prudent to mark more than one site if the exact surgical procedure is in question, such as with a site for a temporary transverse colostomy and a permanent 'end' colostomy in cases where the surgeon is planning to attempt an anterior resection. In such cases the nurse must ensure that the patient fully understands the reason for the double marking and appreciates that this is to provide an alternative for the surgeon, otherwise he may fear he will be left with two stomas.

CRITERIA FOR CHOOSING A STOMA SITE

To ensure secure, leakproof bonding of the appliance to the patient's abdomen, the stoma must be situated on a reasonably smooth, planar body surface.[4] The appliance should cause the patient no discomfort and should not impede his activities. 'A well-sited stoma should enhance movement, deportment and rehabilitation allowing considerable athletic ability.'[5] (See Fig. 36.)

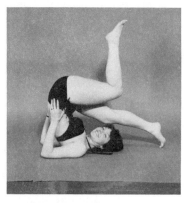

Fig. 36. *A properly sited stoma allows the patient freedom of movement.*

POSSIBLE EFFECTS OF A WRONGLY SITED STOMA (See Fig. 37)

1. The appliance may not bond securely and leakage could occur, resulting in skin excoriation, psychological trauma and curtailment of activities.
2. The patient may not be able to see his stoma, making it impossible for him to execute his own stoma care. This will result in a loss of independence and possibly psychological problems.
3. Activities at work may displace the appliance or cause discomfort; this may prohibit the patient from resuming his employment, producing psychological repercussions and economic connotations.
4. The appliance may prohibit the patient wearing certain styles of clothing, either due to discomfort or because the appliance is conspicuous under some garments. The ability to wear

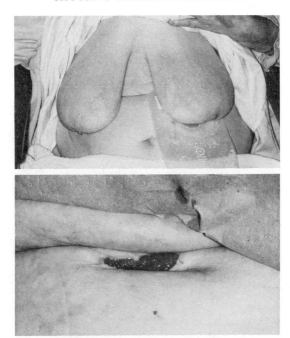

Fig. 37. *Incorrectly placed stomas.*

attractive and stylish clothes is important to many of us, most particularly during teenage years. How sad if a teenager has to wear loose trousers and even braces because his ileostomy is in line with his trouser waistband.

5. The patient's clothing may put pressure on the stoma (for instance a waistband) and result in trauma or leakage.
6. Activity during sports and hobbies may displace the appliance making it impossible for the patient to resume his previous pastimes, for example the keen golfer whose social life revolves around the golf club will be deeply distressed if his golf swing dislodges his appliance. This will curtail not only his sporting activities but also his social life. This can result in psychological frustration or resentment and possible social isolation.

These factors may make the resumption of previous lifestyle impossible for the patient, producing serious psychological repercussions. This will, undoubtedly, affect his rehabilitation and his ability to accept and adjust to having a stoma.

USUAL STOMA SITES

The ileostomy

'The ideal site is on the summit of the infra-abdominal mound over the lower rectus muscle.'[7]

The site for an ileostomy is usually on the right of the abdomen overlying the outer third of the rectus muscle. (See Fig. 38.) It is possible to raise an ileostomy on the left side of the abdomen in cases where a suitable site on the right cannot be found, however this is technically more difficult for the surgeon.

The ileostomy is usually positioned at a point one-third to halfway along a line from the umbilicus to the anterior superior iliac spine.

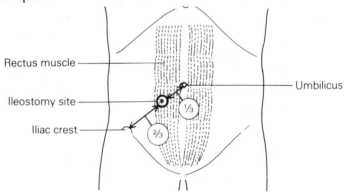

Fig. 38. *Usual site for an ileostomy.*

The 'iliac' or 'end' colostomy

'The pre-operative siting of a colostomy may not be felt to be as vitally important as the placement of an ileostomy but trouble taken can minimize future complications.'[8]

Others would argue against the above opinion, that accurate placement of all stomas is essential to facilitate full rehabilitation. 'The colostomy should be placed on the left of the abdomen so that the emergent bowel penetrates the rectus muscle, rather than the oblique flank muscle.'[9]

The colostomy is usually positioned at a point about one third to halfway along a line from the umbilicus to the anterior superior iliac spine. (See Fig. 39.)

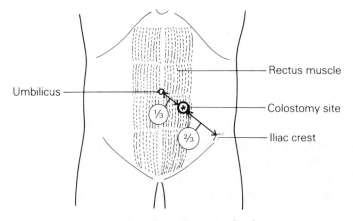

Fig. 39. *Usual site for an iliac or 'end' colostomy.*

The ilial conduit (urostomy)

The ilial conduit is positioned as for the ileostomy. However, in cases when the patient is suffering from spina bifida the stoma must be placed much higher, even above the waist so that it is still visible and does not disappear from view due to a patient's slumped posture if he is in a wheelchair. In some cases it may be advantageous to position a high ileal conduit centrally.

The transverse colostomy

This is most commonly a loop colostomy and is positioned in the right upper abdomen, midway between the costal margin and the

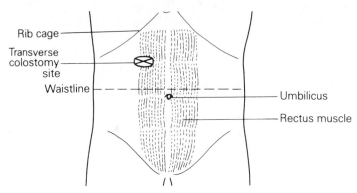

Fig. 40. *Usual site for a transverse colostomy.*

umbilicus in the line of the rectus abdominus muscle.[10] The exact position is determined by finding the most suitable (flat) site. A rough guide would be approximately 5–8 cm below the lower rib cage and 5–8 cm to the right of the umbilicus in the slender candidate. (See Fig. 40.)

STAGES IN ESTABLISHING A SUITABLE STOMA SITE

It is important to explain to the patient each stage in the procedure for siting the stoma and gain his co-operation. He should understand the reasons why the site is chosen preoperatively and the importance of accurate placement.

Stage 1: nursing assessment

Prior to choosing a site to place a stoma, it is essential to know the patient well as an individual. While compiling a nursing history the following information is most pertinent:

- What physical ability does the patient have? Can he stoop, bend, twist and stretch?
- Is the patient's eyesight satisfactory? Does he need spectacles? Can he see his abdomen clearly when he looks down?
- What is the patient's occupation and what exactly is involved? What position does he need to adopt at work (e.g. stretching or crouching)?
- What are his hobbies and interests? Does he participate in any sports? It is important to understand what the hobby/sport involves with regard to movements and posture.
- What is the patient's preference with regard to style of clothing. Does he prefer fitted clothes? It is essential to know the position of the waistband on skirts/trousers. It is also helpful to know what style and type of underwear the patient favours.
- Does the patient depend upon any type of prosthesis (e.g. calliper), and if so what is the position of straps and fittings?
- Does the patient undertake any other particular activity which may influence the stoma site?
- Does the patient have any anxieties or questions regarding the position of the stoma?
- What is the patient's culture? This is particularly pertinent if dealing with members of the Muslim faith whose religion

requires prayers five times daily. This involves the patient crouching forward facing Mecca (the Sujud) and also ritual cleansing prior to prayer. It is worth while to note that if a stoma is placed above the waistline the effluent may be associated with the upper gastrointestinal tract and thus be more acceptable. Effluent from a stoma below the waistline will be classed as dirty and will necessitate the patient cleansing his stoma and changing the appliance prior to each of the five daily prayer sessions.[11] Some Asian cultures use the right hand for preparing and eating foods and other 'clean' purposes, while the left hand is used for body cleansing and other 'dirty' activities. This should be borne in mind when determining the site for a stoma.[12]

Discussion with a surgeon as to exactly what surgical procedure he plans to perform and the type of stoma he intends to fashion is essential. The position of the incision is also pertinent, as is the type of incision the surgeon intends to make. This information must be established, so that the stoma is not placed in too close proximity to the wound.

Stage 2: examine the abdomen and establish physique

Once the nursing assessment is complete the next stage is to examine the patient's abdomen and assess his physique. The

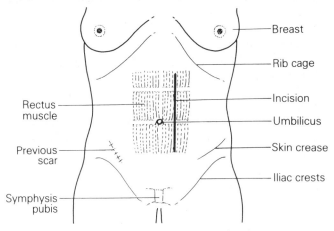

Fig. 41. *Anatomical features to identify.*

patient should be asked to lie semirecumbent, sit forward and stand, during which time the following anatomical features should be identified and avoided when siting the stoma (Fig. 41).

Anatomical features to avoid

- Bony prominences—iliac crests, symphesis pubis, rib cage.
- Natural waistline.
- Skin creases and folds.
- Umbilicus.
- Breasts.
- Previous scars and proposed incision site.
- Any other irregularity in the contours of the abdominal wall.

The stoma must be sited away from these encumbrances as they will impair uncomplicated fitting of a secure collecting appliance. The patient's general physique should also be considered and the position of the rectus muscle envisioned. It should be remembered that the patient may gain or lose weight or, in the case of a child, grow.

Stage 3: choosing a provisional site

After considering the points previously discussed and envisaging the anatomical features to be avoided, a small mark should be made at the proposed site. The patient should then be asked to stand and look down at his abdomen to establish whether he can see this mark; and the site adjusted until it is visible to the patient while standing, since this is the most likely position he will adopt when dealing with his appliance (Fig. 42). The patient should then be asked to move into various other positions to check that the site still appears appropriate.

When a suitable prospective site is chosen an appliance—preferably containing 100 ml of water—should be fitted over the site and the patient should be encouraged to be as active as possible.[13] He should adopt any positions that he may encounter during his daily activities (e.g. crouching, twisting, stooping and bending). He should practice his golf swing, tennis strokes or dancing (if appropriate), as well as sleeping in the appliance. This activity is of the utmost importance and the patient should be

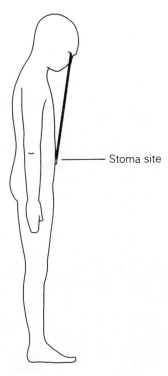

Stoma site

Fig. 42. *Stoma site visible when standing.*

encouraged not to be self-conscious and should be left in privacy, perhaps in the bathroom, to test the site thoroughly. The patient should also dress in his usual clothing while the appliance is *in situ*. This procedure must be coupled with sensitive preoperative counselling as the patient is often very anxious. Great diplomacy must be employed when introducing the patient to appliances for the first time since this can be very distressing if the patient is inadequately prepared psychologically.

Stage 4: evaluation of site

After thoroughly testing the site the outcome should be discussed with the patient to assess whether the appliance has remained comfortable and secure throughout all his activities. It may be that a slightly different site would prove preferable.

Stage 5: marking the site

Once it has been established that the chosen site is suitable, it should be marked with an indelible pen. The patient and nursing staff should be asked to observe the mark to ensure it is not removed during washing or preoperative skin preparation.

If the site chosen is in any way unusual, e.g. high to enable an obese patient to see the stoma, then this should be discussed with the surgeon.

It can be advantageous to site the stoma prior to admission while visiting the patient at home preoperatively. This allows the patient to wear an appliance in his usual surroundings and carry out daily activities; he can actually go out and work in the garden to check that the appliance does not dislodge or dig in.

Emergency cases

In emergency cases it is not possible to follow through all the stages of this procedure. The patient is ill, often in pain and the abdomen may be distended, which will prohibit a full procedure. However, it is still worth while for an experienced person to mark a site preoperatively using her skills of abdominal assessment as the patient may still be able to adopt various postures and the intraoperative problems previously discussed are avoided.

Movement may be limited and distension may be distorting, in which case the site must be marked as appropriately as possible. The surgeon who is faced with the prospect of raising a stoma without a previously marked site for guidance faces several problems. While he will, undoubtedly, have a full knowledge of the patient's medical history and condition, he may only have a very limited knowledge of the patient as an individual. He may thus be unable to give consideration to hobbies, occupation and clothing preferences.

The problem is compounded since the patient is lying flat on a theatre couch, which makes a suitable placement very difficult as the physique changes considerably when the patient is supine. What appears to be a suitable position may disappear beneath a protruding paunch when the patient is standing, or be obstructed from view by pendulous breasts. The effects of muscle relaxant drugs also change the abdominal contours significantly, making it impossible to assess the patient's true shape. In such a situation, when it is not possible to ask the patient to adopt various positions to elicit if skin creases become apparent on movement, the surgeon faces an unenviable task in eliciting a suitable stoma site. It must also be remembered that in some cases the surgeon may find it impossible to position the stoma in the ideal site due to technical constraints in which case the most desirable achievable site should be chosen.

Time spent choosing an accurate stoma site preoperatively is very worth while. Not only does it save nursing time postoperatively, but, more importantly, it can save the patient much discomfort and restriction of activity. The accurate placement of a stoma plays a vital role in the postoperative rehabilitation of the patient and his physical and psychological well-being.

The time to move the position of a stoma is before it is created; this can avoid psychological trauma and physical suffering resulting in the possibility of further surgery for refashioning.

REFERENCES

1. Hughes, E.S.R., Cuthbertson, A.M. & Killingbeck, M.K. (1983) *Colorectal Surgery*. Chap. 12, p.108. Churchill Livingstone.
2. Foulkes, B. (1981) The practical management of bowel stomas. *Stoma Care*, Chap. 4, p. 58. Ed. Breckman, B. Beaconsfield: Beaconsfield.
3. Todd, I. (1978) *Intestinal Stomas* Chap. 7, p.66. London: Heinemann.
4. May, H.J. (1977) *Enterostomal Therapy*, Chap. 13, p.128. New York: Raven Press.
5. Devlin, H.B. (1982a) Coloproctology No 4. In *Stoma Therapy Review II*. p.258.
6. Devlin, H.B. (1982b) Coloproctology No 5. In *Stoma Therapy Review II*, p.298.
7. Devlin, H.B. (1982c) Coloproctology No 4. In *Stoma Therapy Review II*, p.253.
8. Todd, I. (1978) *Intestinal Stomas*, Chap. 1, p.2. London: Heinemann.
9. Devlin, H.B. (1982) Coloproctology No 5. In *Stoma Therapy Review II*, p.298.
10. Todd, I. (1978) *Intestinal Stomas*, Chap 2, p.18. London: Heinemann.
11. Breckman, B. (1981) Psychosocial areas related to stoma care. *Stoma Care* Chap 1, p.1. Ed. Breckman, B. London: Beaconsfield.
12. Henly, A. (1979) *Asian Patients in Hospital and At Home*, Chap. 4, p.47. King Edwards Hospital Fund. London: Pitman Medical.
13. Goligher, J.C. (1984) *Surgery of the Anus, Rectum and Colon*, 5th edn. Chap. 22, p.860. London: Baillière Tindall.

10 Postoperative stoma care

In the immediate postoperative period the patient relies upon the nursing staff to meet his needs and take care of him. Once he begins to recuperate the nurses can involve him in his own care, teaching and encouraging him to become independent once more. However, the patient may resist this independence in an effort to avoid having to accept the stoma.

During this time comes the realization that the stoma is actually there and an alteration in the way he sees his body. This will, ultimately, alter his self-concept and may evoke a variety of psychological responses which are discussed in Chapter 5. The patient does not only have to come to terms with the change in his bodily appearance and function. Now that the stoma is a reality he needs to learn to care for it to enable him to regain a measure of independence which helps to boost self-esteem. He also needs to know what effect the stoma will have on his everyday activities, such things as diet, clothing, personal hygiene and communication.

The change in body image, loss of control over elimination of bodily waste and the need to learn stoma care skills make a tremendous demand on the patient's ability to adapt.

Doering and La Mountain[1,2] have defined postoperative nursing action by designing flow charts to facilitate caring for patients with stomas. These can be very helpful when planning nursing care. This chapter discusses the nursing objectives in the postoperative period and considers how these objectives can be achieved.

POSTOPERATIVE NURSING AIMS AND OBJECTIVES

- Monitor the condition of the stoma and its function.
- Ensure a suitable, comfortable, leakproof appliance is fitted to contain effluent.
- Supply a stock of appliances and accessories for use.
- Encourage the patient to look at the stoma and accept its existence.

- Discuss the outcome of surgery with the patient; encourage him to discuss his prognosis with the medical staff.
- Teach the patient to care for his stoma and the surrounding skin.
- Instruct the patient in methods of draining and changing the appliance.
- Ensure the patient is able to manage his stoma and cope with unforeseen events such as leakage.
- Make the patient aware of how to dispose of appliances in an acceptable manner.
- Explain dietary principles to the patient; ensure he is aware of what foods may result in alteration in stoma function.
- Provide opportunities for counselling and confidential discussion of problems; explore potential problem areas.
- Help the patient select an appliance which is suitable to his individual needs.
- Inform the patient of how to obtain future supplies of appliances and accessories.
- Explain to the patient how to obtain and use a prescription exemption certificate.
- Discuss and assess suitable styles of clothing; build confidence in appearance.
- Explain to the patient any restrictions in his activity during his convalescence.
- Inform the patient what help and support is available after discharge and how this may be obtained.
- Ensure that the patient is in possession of all the information he requires prior to discharge.

It is important that the stoma is closely monitored after surgery. The nurse should check the colour of the stoma while making other routine postoperative observations. The stoma should be the healthy viable reddish-pink colour of mucosa, (similar to the inside of the lower lip). If it appears dusky purple or very dark the medical staff should be informed. The nurse should also check that the appliance has been correctly selected and fitted so that it is not constricting the blood supply to the stoma or causing pressure in any way.

The appliance used in the postoperative period must be made from clear odour-proof plastic to facilitate easy observation of the stoma without its removal. A drainable bag is most suitable for postoperative use because when the stoma starts to function it usually expels loose watery stools. To select the correct size of appliance the nurse should measure the stoma using a measuring guide and select the size of flange with an aperture slightly (3 mm) larger than the stoma itself. This will prevent constriction of the stoma if oedema occurs. If the opening for the stoma is to be cut out or a skin wafer is being used then the edges of the opening should be 'fringed' by making radial cuts, 2 mm long around the cut edge, as shown in Figure 43. This will allow flexibility to accommodate an increase in stoma size.

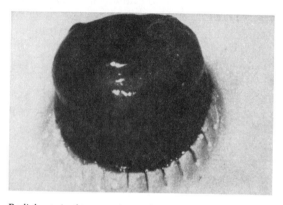

Fig. 43. *Radial cuts in the protective wafer prevent constriction of the stoma.*

In the immediate postoperative period it is unwise to fit a flatus filter to the appliance since it is important to monitor when the patient passes flatus via the stoma. The passage of flatus usually indicates that peristalsis has returned to the intestine and it has recovered from being handled during surgery. A filter may result in the flatus escaping unnoticed from the pouch.

Once a suitable appliance has been selected and fitted a stock of similar equipment should be placed in the patient's own locker. This has two advantages over keeping stock for ward use in a central cupboard: first, the patient has the security of knowing that there is a supply of suitable equipment readily available for his use; and, second, any nurse involved in the patient's care will use appliances from this individual stock if a change is needed, thus ensuring that the patient is always fitted with a suitable appliance.

The nurse should monitor and record the passage of flatus and the volume and nature of the effluent. It is essential that the appliance is not allowed to become overfull, since this will make it very heavy and the weight may compromise the adhesion resulting in leakage. The nurses will be responsible for caring for the stoma and appliance until the patient is well enough to learn self-care. Talking through the procedures as they are carried out can be a good basis for future teaching. However, it must be remembered that not all the information given will be retained.

The patient may need encouragement and support to enable him to look at his stoma for the first time. This can be a traumatic experience and the nurse should be sensitive to the patient's feelings. It is vital that the nurse does not show any sign of revulsion by word or gesture when dealing with the stoma as the patient will be scrutinizing her responses closely. Any sign of distaste, however small, will be used by the patient to reinforce his fears of being unacceptable.

The patient and his family will be anxious to know the outcome of the operation and will seek reassurance regarding his progress. It is important that the nurse answers any questions raised honestly and demonstrates a positive attitude towards the patient's condition and progress. However, the nurse should not offer false or premature reassurance. The patient should have the opportunity to discuss his prognosis and future treatment if he wishes to and should be encouraged to voice his questions. The nurse may need to act as 'patient's advocate' if he feels unable to discuss his treatment with medical staff. It is vital that all the member of the caring team give the patient the same information to avoid possible confusion. Members of the patient's family should be involved in promoting a positive attitude. They should be encouraged to demonstrate their acceptance of the patient and to act normally towards him. Family support can be vital to the patient's rehabilitation; it is helpful to warn the patient's family that he may test them out and will be observing their responses and actions closely for any sign of non-acceptance or distaste.

Once the patient is more alert, teaching can begin to enable him to care for his own stoma. Henderson states 'Patient teaching is an inherent part of nursing as well as an innate patient right'.[3] In her model for nursing care Orem[4] sees nurses as being concerned with an individual's needs and ability to perform self-care to sustain health, to recover from disease or injury or to cope with the effects of disease or injury. If a patient is taught to meet the additional demands placed on his self-care capabilities by having a stoma, then a balance is established and nursing is not required, thus the patient regains his independence.

Teaching cannot usually be effective until about the third or fourth postoperative day and then practical skills will be limited if the patient's arm is immobilized due to an intravenous infusion. Prior to this, the patient will probably retain little information because of the effects of anaesthesia and analgesia coupled with postoperative discomfort. Anxiety can also be a barrier to learning. 'Retention of information is poor when patients are preoccupied with anxieties about their illness and its effects. Anxious patients commonly deny having been given information or teaching when it has definitely been given.'[5] It is therefore important for the nurse to try and relieve the patient's anxiety as much as possible, by providing support, offering reassurance and explaining the patient's treatment to him, and ensuring that he is aware of what to expect.

Prior to commencing teaching the nurse should have a clear plan of what she hopes to achieve. She should decide upon her objectives and then establish a series of achievable goals. Ideally the patient shoud be involved in the goal-setting process since this will be more conducive to achievement. These objectives will enable the nurse to evaluate critically the patient's performance and measure the effectiveness of her teaching. However, the nurse must consider the mental and physical ability of the individual patient and accept that there are those who will never be able to achieve self-care.

Aim

Prior to discharge from hospital the patient will be able to carry out an appliance change correctly without aid.

Teaching objectives

After the teaching sessions the patient will be able to:

- Identify the equipment required to perform an appliance change.

- Prepare an appliance correctly prior to changing.
- Empty a drainable appliance and demonstrate the correct use of the clip.
- Remove a soiled appliance demonstrating the learned technique.
- Cleanse and dry the skin surrounding the stoma, demonstrating the application of any necessary skin protectives.
- Measure the stoma to ensure that the appliance used is the correct size.
- Correctly fit a new appliance.
- Apply an appliance cover.
- Demonstrate the use of any accessories, e.g. a belt.
- Dispose of soiled appliance in an acceptable manner.

Before teaching begins the nurse should create an environment conducive to learning by:

- Providing privacy.
- Eliminating distractions.
- Minimizing interruptions.

The nurse should also be aware of the basic principles that will enable her to teach effectively. It is helpful to break down the skill to be taught into each component action as this will aid logical and clear explanation.

Teaching principles

- Make the patient feel at ease.
- Assess the patient's learning needs.
- Use language that the patient is familiar with and can easily understand, avoiding jargon or abbreviations.
- Establish the need for learning; give reasons why the procedure is necessary.
- Do not assume prior knowledge; ask questions to establish previous learning.
- State objectives, explain clearly the skill to be taught.
- Demonstrate skill to patient.
- Allow the patient to practise the required skill; do not rush patient by word or gesture.
- Reinforce desired performance.
- Correct mistakes diplomatically.

- Do not give too much information at any one time.
- Encourage the patient to ask questions.
- Obtain feedback of learning by asking the patient to repeat or demonstrate what he has been taught.

The information that is given to the patient should be organized into a logical sequence but must remain flexible to enable the nurse to deal with questions as they arise and teach accordingly.

Teaching plan

Teach use of clip and method of emptying appliance

Use of deodorant spray may help alleviate odour that can be distressing to the patient, particularly if he is nauseated. The patient may be given a clean bag and clip so that he can practise the technique repeatedly. In this way any mistake will not result in leaks or spills that may act as a barrier to future efforts.

Once this skill has been mastered the patient should be encouraged to empty his own appliance under supervision, since this will give him a sense of achievement and restore a degree of independence. Those patients with an iliac colostomy who will eventually use a closed appliance should still be taught this skill in case at any time they develop diarrhoea and need to use a drainable appliance.

Teach preparation of appliance

The preparation of the appliance that is required will vary depending upon make and design. Teaching should again be divided into stages, which may include marking and cutting out a flange or skin wafer, application of a flatus patch and use of deodorizing powder.

Once the relevant stage has been taught the patient should be allowed to practise alone. For example, he could be asked to mark and cut out the flange in preparation for the next appliance change. This provides the nurse with feedback as to the success of the tuition as well as being positive reinforcement for the patient, it makes him feel useful and appreciate that he is learning.

Changing the appliance

When the patient is adept at the preparation of his appliance he should be taught to change the bag.

Gloves should not be worn when dealing with the stoma as 'skin-to-skin' contact shows the patient that the nurse accepts the stoma and peristomal skin, helping to integrate them into a new body image. Patients frequently feel that they must be 'dirty' if the nurse wears gloves when caring for the stoma.[6]

The technique of removing the appliance and disposal should be explained and demonstrated. The patient should then be shown how to cleanse and dry the peristomal skin and apply a skin protective if one is to be used. The patient should practise these procedures under supervision at future appliance changes until the technique is mastered. The patient must be shown how to measure his stoma and identify the correct size of appliance. He can then be taught to fit a clean appliance. The precise fitting technique will vary depending upon the make and type of appliance being used. It may be necessary to change the appliance more frequently during this learning period to provide the patient with opportunities to practise. However, the nurse must make sure the patient is aware of the correct frequency for routine changing.

Use of accessories

When the patient is capable of changing his appliance he should be taught the use of any accessories he needs, such as belts, tape, etc.

While teaching should always take place in stages, it is helpful to describe all the stages of the procedure as they are performed, emphasizing the particular technique being taught and concentrating upon this. The patient should be encouraged to ask questions and the nurse should obtain feedback of her tuition by asking the patient to repeat what he has been told or demonstrate what he has learned. Once he is capable, the patient should be encouraged to change his appliance alone in privacy and the application should then be checked. The ward bathroom is the ideal place to change the appliance once the patient is ambulant as it facilitates privacy and is probably most like the place where changing will take place at home.

It is essential to ensure that the patient has carried out at least one appliance change alone and unaided prior to discharge. If the patient is not capable of this then the person who is to assist at home should be involved prior to the patient leaving the ward to ensure continuity of care.

It is helpful if a close relative is able to change the appliance in case the patient himself is ever incapacitated. The teaching of this person is better postponed until the patient himself is competent. He can then demonstrate the technique to his relative with a nurse present, and this will act as a reinforcement for the patient who gains a sense of achievement from airing his knowledge. If the nurse teaches a relative before the patient is competent there is a danger that the patient will cease trying to learn, putting the responsibility of care onto his loved one which may prove impractical or become a burden. Another danger is that the relative may learn more quickly than the patient who has undergone surgery and this can be frustrating for him, making him feel inadequate.

Some patients may benefit from being given a written instruction sheet to aid their memory of the stages involved in changing their appliance; an example is given below. The points made should be clear and concise and not cluttered with too much detail. It is essential, however, that such a list does not take the place of teaching—it must only act as a learning aid.

EXAMPLE OF PATIENT'S INSTRUCTION SHEET

1. Collect all equipment together, i.e. appliance and accessories, skin protective, measuring guide, bowl of warm water, kitchen paper, rubbish bag, newspaper.
2. Spread newspaper for rubbish.
3. Ensure new appliance is prepared.
4. Empty bag.
5. Gently remove bag, peeling from the top downwards.
6. Cleanse skin around stoma with plain warm water.
7. Dry skin well.
8. Measure stoma to check correct appliance size.
9. Apply skin protective.
10. Fit new bag.
11. Check bag is secure and correctly fitted.
12. Check clip is secure.
13. Wrap all soiled items well in newspaper and put into plastic bag prior to disposal in the dustbin.

The post-operative period is often an uncertain time and there may be instances of leakage or spills occurring in the ward. The nurse should take this opportunity to teach the patient how to cope with the incident. While he should be reassured that accidents or leaks rarely occur if he is wearing a suitable and correctly applied appliance, it is important that he can cope with the situation and act accordingly. If there are no mishaps while he is in hospital the patient should be warned that a leak could occur and the possible causes of this discussed. He should also be advised as to the action to take if leakage persists.

While he is in hospital the patient should be given the information he needs to prepare him for coping with his stoma at home.

Disposing of soiled appliances

Disposal of soiled appliances is a question that worries many patients. Burning on an open fire should be discouraged because the plastic may give off harmful fumes when heated. If the patient has a closed, solid fuel boiler then he may wish to dispose of appliances by burning. Few patients will have this facility and, consequently, patients can be advised to empty the soiled appliance and wrap it well in newspaper; it should then be put into a plastic bag and disposed of into the dustbin. Most local authorities operate a soiled dressing collection service whereby the patient disposes of his soiled appliance into a plastic bag supplied by the authority and a van calls, usually once a week, to make a collection. However, stoma patients frequently decline this service as they feel that the special collection may draw attention from neighbours and result in attached stigma.

Special Comex disposal units are available which consist of a blue box container with a dispenser for aromatic germicide built into the lid. The patient puts his soiled appliance into the container and a small amount of germicide is automatically dispensed into the box by closing the lid. These containers are delivered and collected by the company regularly, or alternatively the container may be collected with the normal refuse. Emptying of the appliances prior to disposal is said to be unnecessary by the manufacturer, Cannon Hygiene Ltd. Some patients find this method of disposal very acceptable while others dislike the thought of soiled appliances being kept so long or find the unit too conspicuous. There is a charge for this unit which includes delivery; in some areas this cost may be met by the local authority.

When travelling, appliances can be disposed of in a similar manner to that used at home or patients may be able to obtain specially designed disposable bags for use when travelling. One or two appliance companies supply such bags free of charge to customers. Others are available for purchase from some stoma suppliers. Once the empty appliance is sealed into a disposal bag it can be discarded in a rubbish bin. Some female patients use sanitary towel incinerators in ladies toilets.

Diet

The patient will require information regarding his diet since he may not be aware of the foods that could cause alteration in stomal function. He should be advised to eat a varied and balanced diet, experimenting with new foods in small quantities. If the patient experiences a problem with odour, flatulence or loose motions he should take a note of the foods he has eaten in the previous 24 hours. In this manner he should be able to identify the trigger of his problems. The patient must then decide whether his pleasure from eating a particular food is worth the after-effects. If it is a favourite food he may well decide to eat it and cope with the consequences. However, he should be advised to ensure that he only eats such food when he has easy access to a lavatory to cope with possible problems. Further information regarding dietary considerations for stoma patients is given in Chapter 16.

The nurse should provide the patient with opportunity to voice his anxieties and discuss his problems. The patient's questions must be answered honestly, avoiding false or premature reassurance. It is often helpful to the patient if the nurse can facilitate exploration of potential problem areas. Research suggests that postoperative counselling of stoma patients who had cancer results in a positive alteration in self-concept/self-esteem.[7,9]

Appliances

If the patient has been shown a selection of appliances in the preoperative period he may have stated a preference for a particular type or style of bag. Once regular inspection of the stoma is no longer necessary the patient may prefer to use an opaque appliance. If the patient has an 'end' colostomy he will usually progress to using a 'closed' type of appliance once his motion is formed. The patient should be encouraged to select an appliance that is suitable to his individual needs. The nurse may need to offer guidance as there is such a wide variety of products, each with different features and benefits. The patient's type of stoma, physique and lifestyle should be considered when assessing the suitability of individual appliances. The patient may wish to try several different products to satisfy himself that he is using the one most suitable for him. If this is the case he should select one appliance to use until he is adept in caring for his stoma and changing the bag. Once he has established a routine of stoma care and is at home he can then experiment with other products until he makes his final choice. Further information about stoma care appliances and accessories is given in Chapter 4.

Prior to leaving hospital the patient should be given a stock of appliances and equipment to last until he has obtained a further supply in the community. It is usually necessary to give patients 2–3 weeks' supply of stock to take home, since following discharge he must reorientate himself at home, see a doctor and obtain a prescription. The prescription is then taken to a retail pharmacist in the usual way but the equipment usually needs to be ordered as there is too great a variety for the chemist to stock all types, and delivery time on stock varies. If the patient has an adequate supply the fear of running out of equipment is removed.

The patient should also be given a list of prescription requisites which specifies the appliance and accessories being used. This information about the products should include:

- The make.
- The type.
- The size.
- The manufacturer's code number.
- The pack size.
- The approximate quantity to last one month.

A copy of these prescription details should also be supplied to the patient's general practitioner and pharmacist.

It is helpful if the patient uses the same pharmacy regularly as he can then establish a relationship with the pharmacist who will often keep a small amount of equipment in stock for regular customers. Some pharmacists are particularly helpful to stoma patients and establish a local reputation; some may provide a delivery service for frail or elderly patients.

Prescriptions can also be dealt with by mail order; there are several appliance distributors who will dispatch stoma care products promptly by post on receipt of a prescription. Some patients prefer to use such a service, finding it more discreet than regular visits to the local chemists.

Patients who have a permanent stoma are exempt from prescription charges. Exemption is obtained by completing Form P11 from the post office. The appropriate section of the form stating that the patient has a permanent fistula which requires an appliance is then completed and signed by the patient. The form must be countersigned by the patient's general practitioner or hospital doctor prior to being sent to the local family practitioner committee office. The patient will then receive an exemption certificate valid for three years. This procedure should be explained to the patient and he may need to be shown how to complete the back of the prescription form (FP10) once he is in possession of his certificate.

Clothing

The patient may be apprehensive about dressing in his outdoor clothing. It is often when dressing prior to discharge that the reality of the stoma becomes most apparent. Night attire may have been associated with hospital and a protected environment, while dressing in outdoor clothing may bring about an awareness in the patient that he is to go out and face the world with his altered body image.

The nurse should discuss preference in styles of clothing with the patient and providing that the stoma has been accurately placed he can be told there should be little restriction in choice. Some patients like to wear firm corsets which may be uncomfortable after surgery—they may also apply pressure on the stoma which can result in leakage or damage to the stoma. These patients should be advised not to wear their corsets initially. Once they find wearing a firm support comfortable, a fitting can be arranged for a 'stoma girdle'. These have an appropriately placed opening to avoid pressure on the stoma or leakage. Patients are entitled to two such corsets on prescription each year. If the patient likes to wear stockings rather than tights these should be held up by a suspender belt or the patient may prefer to buy stockings with elastic tops, provided she has no circulatory problems.

The patient may well need time to rebuild confidence in his appearance. It may prove helpful for him to have some clothes brought into the ward so that he can dress and reassure himself that the stoma is not detectable under clothing. The patient may benefit from having a nurse present to offer support when he dresses for the first time. He should be encouraged to try different types and styles of clothing to ascertain if any particular design presents a problem. The patient should be discouraged from restricting himself to baggy, loose clothing, unless he usually finds this type of dress preferable. Once the patient has worn normal clothing for a day or two he usually realizes that nobody notices he is any different since the appliance is not detectable, and this will help boost his confidence.

Convalescence

Many patients are unsure of what activities are restricted during their convalescence. The nurse should explain to the patient what to avoid and why. The stoma itself poses little problem, it is the fact that the patient has undergone abdominal surgery that is the restricting factor. Thus the advice given to the patient regarding resumption of physical activities is the same as that for any other patient who has undergone major abdominal surgery.

Prior to leaving the ward the patient should be told what support is available to him when he is at home. He should be given the name, address and telephone number of the nurse he should contact if he experiences any problems with his stoma. If there is a nurse specialist available to visit him at home then she should liaise with the community nurse to provide continuity of care. If there is no nurse specialist to liaise it is important that the community nurse is given adequate information from the hospital to enable her to continue the patient's care and avoid giving conflicting advice which may cause confusion. It is ideal if the community nurse can meet the patient in the ward before he leaves hospital so that a relationship can be established.

It is essential that the patient is given all the information he needs to ensure that his transition from hospital to home is accomplished smoothly without fear or anxiety. Patient teaching is a major responsibility of the nursing staff to ensure that his information needs are met. Without adequate knowledge and preparation for discharge, patients may feel nervous and unable to cope with their recovery at home.[8]

The patient should be told when he can expect to be visited at home by a nurse and encouraged to telephone for help or advice if he needs any.

REFERENCES

1. Doering, K.J. & La Mountain, P. (1984) Flow charts to facilitate caring for ostomy patients. Part 2 *Nursing*, October, 47–49.
2. Doering, K.J. & La Mountain, P. (1984) Flow charts to facilitate caring for ostomy patients. Part 3 *Nursing* November, 54–57.
3. Henderson, V. (1961) *Basic Principles of Nursing Care*. International Council of Nurses, Geneva. 38–41.
4. Orem, D. (1980) *Nursing: Concepts of Practice*. New York: McGraw Hill.
5. Webb, P. (1985) Getting it right—patient teaching. *Nursing* Vol.2, No.38 June 2, 1125–1127.
6. Wilson, W. & Desriusseaux, B. (1983) Stoma care and patient teaching. *Patient Teaching*. Ed. Wilson Barnett, J. London: Churchill Livingstone, Chap. 6, 95–118.
7. Watson, P.G. (1983) The effects of short term post-operative counselling on cancer/ostomy patients. *Cancer Nursing*, February, 21–29.
8. Wilson Barnett, J. (1985) Principles of patient teaching. *Nursing Times* 20 February, 28–29.
9. Watson, P.G. (1983) Post-operative counselling for cancer/ostomy patients. *Journal of Enterostomal Therapy, 10*, May/June 84–91.

11   Community aspects of stoma care

When the patient leaves the protected environment of the hospital where help and support are available throughout the 24-hour period, he may feel very insecure. He faces the problems of readaptation into the community, resumption of his previous lifestyle and reintegration into his family unit.[1]

'Even with good pre-operative counselling and effective practical teaching of basic stoma care, many patients do not fully realise the true impact of stoma surgery until they have been discharged from hospital.'[2]

Research indicates that stoma patients may encounter a variety of problems when they return to the community.[3,4] These may include difficulties with the use of the appliance, resulting in leakage, odour and sore skin. The patient may have inadequate or inconvenient sanitary facilities at home which can compound his problem, or there may be difficulty in obtaining and disposing of stoma care equipment. Life with a stoma demands adaptation and changes in ingrained habits of personal hygiene.

Problems may also occur for the patient in relating to his family and friends, worrying about their reaction towards him and fearing rejection. This can result in curtailed social and recreational activities, possibly leading to social isolation. Emotional problems may occur due to changed body image leading to poor self-concept and low self-esteem. These feelings may manifest in a variety of psychological responses, such as projected anger, denial or depression. The patient may feel that he is unable to communicate his fears and anxieties to others.

Following major surgery there may be an inability to cope with the activities of daily living which, in turn, creates a further loss of independence for stoma patients. As well as problems of personal hygiene, employment difficulties and sexual dysfunction may also occur. In addition, some patients may develop nutritional deficiences if they place unnecessarily stringent dietary restrictions upon themselves in an attempt to control stoma function.

Once he has been discharged from hospital the patient may experience a temporary loss of self-confidence. On arriving home he may feel anxious and be unsure of his ability to cope with his stoma and resume his previous lifestyle. He will be exposed to his family, friends and neighbours in his normal environment for the first time. This can be a stressful experience as the patient explores reactions towards him.

To enable her to continue the care and support required by the patient after discharge, the nurse who visits him in the community must be in possession of all the relevant information. If the nurse has met the patient while he was in hospital she can build on the relationship she has established with him and his family, to enable her to continue supportive counselling. Once the patient is at home he becomes once again the responsibility of the general practitioner. It is therefore important that any nurse visiting the patient in his own home communicates with the patient's own doctor and informs him of any relevant aspects of the patient's care.

It is advantageous if there is a stoma care nurse who can visit the patient after he goes home. Her role is to liaise with members of the primary health care team to facilitate continuity of care. She should liaise with the community nursing staff who are involved in the patient's care to ensure there is effective use of limited resources and nursing time.

NURSING AIMS AND OBJECTIVES FOR STOMA CARE IN THE COMMUNITY

- Facilitating the smooth transition between hospital and home, thus minimizing possible fear or anxiety.
- Liaising with members of the primary health care team to facilitate effective communication and continuity of care.
- Assessing the patient's ability to cope with activities of daily living.
- Monitoring of family relationships and attitudes, assessment of the patient's reintegration into the family group.
- Ensuring the patient is able to carry out the care of his stoma in his own home.

- Reiterating and expanding the information given in hospital pertaining to practical stoma management.
- Ensuring a prescription for appliances and equipment has been obtained and that supplies are available. Advising the patient about suitable storage for stoma care equipment.
- Helping the patient to adapt to alterations in long-standing habits.
- Continuing supportive counselling; offering emotional support to help facilitate psychological adaptation.
- Recognizing at the onset any specific problems and liaising with the relevant expert who can offer help to the patient, e.g. surgeon, social worker, disablement resettlement officer.
- Assessing the patient's eating habits and advising on nutritional requirements and diet.
- Encouraging the patient to resume recreational, social and sporting activities.
- Counselling the patient with regard to resuming sexual relationships.
- Facilitating the patient's return to gainful employment if appropriate.
- Ensuring the patient is aware of what support is available to him in the community and how to get help and advice if necessary in the future.
- Explaining clinic arrangements for stoma care and surgical follow-up and encouraging the patient to attend.
- Monitoring of rehabilitation; support and encouragement of the patient in the resumption of his previous lifestyle.
- Providing a service of care and support until full rehabilitation is achieved.

Ideally the patient who has a stoma should be visited at home within two days of discharge. When she visits, the nurse should make various observations which will help her to establish how well the patient is readapting. If she has visited the patient at home prior to surgery the information she gained then will provide her with a basis on which to judge the present situation.

Nursing observations

Observation of the general condition of the home may give the nurse clues about possible inability of the patient to cope with household chores. An unkempt house may be a sign that the patient is in need of practical help, or could be a clue to financial hardship. If necessary, the nurse in the community can arrange for the patient to have the benefit of a home-help.

The nurse should observe the patient's general demeanour and how he greets her. Is his personality the same? Have family relationships altered? What is the general atmosphere like within the home? This information will enable her to assess the patient's reintegration into the family group. If there appears to be a fraught, tense atmosphere in the household and the patient is ill at ease or withdrawn, the nurse may have to offer help and support to the family group to enable them to come to terms with the situation. Sometimes members of the family need to express their own anxieties and doubts about having the patient back at home. The nurse may need to encourage the family to demonstrate their acceptance of the patient, explaining that he will be watching for any changes in their attitude towards him now that he has a stoma.

Practical aspects of stoma management

Discussion with the patient regarding his routine for caring for his stoma should elicit any practical problems or difficulties. The appliance application should be checked and the nurse should ensure that the stoma and surrounding skin is healthy. If the patient has encountered any problems in dealing with the stoma in his own home it may be necessary to make practical suggestions regarding modification of his routine or improvising facilities. If toilet and bathroom facilities are inadequate the social services department of the local authority may be able to arrange for the appropriate modifications to be made. Provision of an inside toilet and running water should be considered as a minimum requirement. In more extreme cases the housing department may be persuaded to find alternative accommodation for the patient and his family.

The method of appliance disposal should be ascertained to ensure that the patient is dealing with soiled appliances in an acceptable manner. It may be necessary to arrange for collection of clinical waste by the local authority if the patient wishes it.

Provided that the patient and his general practitioner have been given a comprehensive, accurate list of stoma care requirements the doctor will usually give the patient a prescription for a month's supply of equipment at his first visit. There may be a delay in obtaining these supplies as the pharmacist usually has to place a special order so it is vital that the nurse checks the patient has an adequate supply of equipment to last until his stock arrives. If the patient runs out of equipment he can become very disturbed. He should be advised to obtain a further prescription when he has used half his current supply. Storage may be a problem as most appliances should be kept in a cool place; a spare room that is not heated is usually the most suitable place. The patient should be advised to rotate his stock to avoid keeping appliances for too long prior to use.

Some patients, particularly the elderly, find difficulty coming to terms with changes in their routine of personal hygiene and require practical advice and support to enable them to adapt to new habits. It may be beneficial if stoma care routines are kept as simple as possible to avoid lengthy rituals which can compound the problems of adaptation.

Emotional support

Opportunities to continue supportive counselling should be sought. It is important to identify what the patient's feelings towards having a stoma are now that he is out of hospital and to assess his ability to cope. The anxieties that the patient faced in the postoperative period may well differ from the problems he is now encountering. Initially, practical care is often a major problem but once these procedures have been mastered the patient may become anxious about the more long-term aspects of his rehabilitation, such as resumption of hobbies or sporting activities. If the patient is experiencing emotional problems these may manifest in a variety of psychological reactions, some of which are discussed in Chapter 5.

The nurse should endeavour to enable the patient to talk about his problems and anxieties, helping him to explore his feelings and come to terms with them. If it becomes apparent that the patient is showing signs of severe emotional disturbance which the nurse feels are beyond the scope of her counselling skills, she should acknowledge this. A referral should be sensitively discussed with the patient, making sure that he does not interpret it as a rebuff. The nurse must then seek agreement from the patient's general practitioner to enlist further help. If the patient feels that he has been part of this referral decision he may well co-operate more fully, and thus benefit more, from the help he receives.

There are some areas of care in which the nurse may feel that her expertise is limited, in which case it is vital to obtain a referral to other appropriate professionals from the patient's own doctor. The nurse can then act as a valuable link between these sources of help.

Nutritional advice

Patients who have undergone major surgery on the gastrointestinal tract often find that their appetite is diminished during their convalescence; this is often made worse if the patient is anxious, has emotional problems or is depressed.[5] Patients who have a stoma may severely restrict their dietary intake in the belief that this will curtail stoma function. It is important that diet is discussed fully with the patient to establish what he is eating and if his appetite has changed. Advice may be required regarding meal planning since it is more satisfactory to eat spaced smaller meals rather than one large daily feast. He should be made aware of the foods that may cause an increase in flatus and odour or produce a more fluid stool. Patients with an ileostomy should be warned that foods high in cellulose may cause discomfort or result in obstruction. These foods should be taken in moderation and must be chewed thoroughly. It is, however, equally important to ensure that the patient can still enjoy a varied and nutritionally balanced diet. Patients with a stoma, particularly an ileostomy, should be advised to maintain an adequate fluid intake. (See Chapter 16.)

If the patient's appetite is poor he may need to be tempted with small, attractively served meals. Some patients may find it a problem to prepare a nutritious hot meal when their energy is still impaired following surgery. If this is the case it may be possible to arrange for hot meals to be delivered to the patient two or three times a week by the meals-on-wheels service. Some patients may benefit from nutritional supplements which are taken in addition to meals and can replace possible deficiencies in their diet. Some of these high protein, palatable, easily digested products are prescribable by the doctor for patients who suffer from certain medical conditions.

Stigma

Many stoma patients admit to being aware of a degree of stigma.[6,7] This occurs when an individual is unable to achieve full social or self-acceptance because he sees himself as physically disadvantaged, no longer being 'normal'. Stigma may result in the stoma patient withdrawing from social contact and becoming isolated,[7] and the nurse should be aware of the danger of this if she is to help the patient achieve full rehabilitation.

Resumption of social activities

During her visits to the home the nurse should assess whether or not the patient appears to be resuming his normal activities. If the patient is dressed this is often a sign that he is beginning to adapt to his stoma and has some confidence in the appliance. The patient may require encouragement to resume his recreational interests and hobbies. It may be that the patient is not physically able to participate in sports for a few months but he can still maintain an interest and spectate. Other hobbies are less demanding and can provide a welcome diversion for the patient who is not yet able to undertake more physical pastimes.

Some patients are reluctant to resume their social activities fearing that they will not be accepted now that they have a stoma. If the patient is unwilling to go out and there have been few visitors to the home this may indicate that the patient is anxious and avoiding social contact. These fears must be explored and overcome if full rehabilitation is to be achieved.

To enable the patient to feel able to resume social contact it may be helpful to work with him in establishing a viable plan of action. This will usually involve the patient deciding upon his ultimate aim and then setting himself a series of realistic goals so that the desired outcome is achieved in stages. Each goal that is set should have a time limit by which it should have been achieved. An example of this type of structured counselling is outlined in Chapter 6. The nurse can assist the patient by talking the problems through with him and helping to compile his plan. She should then lend her support by discussing the accomplishment of each goal and evaluating the degree of success achieved. It is essential that the nurse allows the patient to plan his own strategy and set his own goals. This ensures that he is the instigator of the action. He is then more likely to achieve his desired outcome.

Personal relationships

Sexual dysfunction may occur in stoma patients due to physiological or psychological causes. Great tact and diplomacy must be employed by the nurse when she is exploring the patient's resumption of sexual activity. She may be able to help by listening to the patient as he expresses his feelings and explores ways in which he can come to terms with them. Some practical suggestions, such as a change in position for sexual intercourse or the use of an attractive appliance cover may be helpful. Expert help should be sought if the nurse recognizes that the patient's problem is too complex for her to deal with. Many patients will occupy separate beds or even separate rooms when they first leave hospital after major surgery. The reason for this is often that they fear their partner may accidentally injure them when they move around during sleep. This may be acceptable but the nurse should be vigilant as to how long this change in sleeping arrangements persists. If the couple continue to sleep separately then it may indicate an underlying problem in their intimate relationship. Some couples experience difficulty in talking opening to each other about sexual anxieties. They find that they cannot easily express their feelings and doubts in words or they worry that their partner will not be receptive to their fears. The nurse may need to encourage the couple to talk together privately or facilitate such a discussion by being present as a third party and prompting open conversation. If sexual activity is impaired it may be helpful to advise the couple to maintain physical contact and seek alternative methods of gratification.

Employment

The patient should be able to resume his previous employment once he is physically fit; this is usually about 12 weeks after surgery. Some patients, particularly the elderly, may find that they cannot manage the job they were doing prior to their operation and require advice about retraining. However, before recommending that the patient seeks alternative employment it must be established that the patient is not just encountering prejudice because he has a stoma. In many cases this manifests from ignorance on the part of the employer or fellow employees.

Most stoma patients are particularly fastidious in their personal habits and have very high standards of hygiene. 'They can be confidently recommended for classically clean jobs such as consultant surgeon, nurse or bakery worker,' writes consultant surgeon H. Brendan Devlin.[8] He goes on to say: 'Altering the employment of an elderly colostomate may be just another onslaught on his self esteem to which he may be unable to adjust.'[8]

If the patient does encounter problems in returning to work the nurse may be able to offer assistance. This may take the form of practical advice, for instance if a patient with a urostomy is unable to get to the lavatory to empty his appliance regularly he may need to use a urine 'leg-bag' to provide added capacity while at work. If the patient is willing the nurse may be able to talk to the employer and give him more information about life with a stoma. This education may bring about a realization that his prejudice is unjustified. Liaison with the occupational health nurse if there is one may also be fruitful.

Patients who have had an ileostomy for inflammatory bowel disease can expect to achieve a full life expectancy. In fact, once the disease is cured their general health usually improves markedly resulting in more regular attendance at work and increased productivity. If patients do experience employment difficulties then the voluntary stoma associations will give support and advice.

The nurse should make the patient aware of what help and support is available to him in the community. She should explain to the patient the function of the various professionals and voluntary organizations, so that he can recognize the most likely source of help in a particular circumstance. If there is a stoma care nurse she can act as a link between the patient and other available sources of help. It is vital that all stoma patients have someone whom they can contact if they experience difficulties or anxieties after they leave hospital. Information about the sources of help available to stoma patients is given in Chapter 12.

The nurse who has contact with the patient after he leaves hospital should monitor his rehabilitation and encourage and support him in his attempt to resume his previous lifestyle. Support should be continued as long as the patient requires it but the nurse should be alert to the danger of the patient becoming overdependent on her. The relationship between a nurse and the patient with a stoma is often long-standing.

The nurse/patient relationship

The patient may have come to trust and respect the nurse a great deal, particularly if she has been instrumental in helping him to express and overcome some very intimate problems. This can, occasionally, give rise to a transference of affection where the patient at an unconscious level begins to see the nurse as someone very important in his life. This is often someone from his past and particularly occurs if the patient recognizes some similarity between the nurse and a loved one he has lost. The nurse visiting in the home should be alert to this potential danger as the helping relationship may be damaged by a series of imagined problems, frequent calls to attend or an actual physical advance. This situation is best confronted and dealt with by frank discussion with the patient.

It may be helpful if the nurse brings about an awareness in the patient of why this has occurred, asking: 'Do I remind you of someone else?' or 'Do I talk like somebody else?' The problem should be seen as a joint one and it may be more appropriate to use the term 'we'—'*We* appear to have a problem...'. It is also possible for a transference of dislike to occur if the patient recognizes in the nurse traits of another person whom he disliked. This can be equally destructive to a successful nurse/patient relationship.

Conversely the nurse must avoid 'crowding' or 'mothering' the patient. Some individuals learn to look after themselves very quickly and become independent. They may become embarrassed at any fuss or overdiscussion of personal problems. In this situation the nurse should withdraw, allowing the patient his independence but ensuring that he knows how to obtain any help he may need.

Domiciliary visits can be curtailed once the patient is progressing satisfactorily. However, links with the nurse should be maintained, possibly via the stoma care clinic. This helps to ensure that the patient has access to help if it is needed.

Continuing support

The surgeon usually arranges to see the patient in an outpatient clinic. If there is a stoma care nurse available the patient may wish to combine his appointment with an opportunity to see her and discuss any problems. An invitation to telephone or attend the clinic at other times should be extended. If there are alternative stoma care clinics available which the patient can attend, then details of these should be given to the patient. It is often advantageous if the patient has an option of venue or time, particularly if he has resumed work.

It is debatable whether frequent regular attendance at a stoma care clinic is justifiable. Such visits certainly have the advantage of monitoring the patient closely, which should result in early recognition and treatment of problems. However, they may also foster dependence, necessitate regular absences from work and over use limited resources and nursing time. A less formal pattern of clinic attendance is most cost-effective and enables the patient to attend only when he feels it necessary. However, this system places on the patient the onus to seek help. Stoma patients should be encouraged to attend the clinic as often as necessary if they have problems or require advice and support. An annual visit may be helpful in keeping the patient up to date with advances in appliances and equipment. This contact will also allow the nurse the opportunity to monitor discreetly the patient's progress, identify any problems and assess his degree of rehabilitation.

REFERENCES

1. Bontoft, S. (1978) Stoma care in the community. In *Intestinal Stomas*. Ed. Todd, I. Chap.20, pp.168–170. London: Heinemann.
2. Brady, V.A. (1980) Community care of the stoma patient. *Nursing, 17*, 741–743.
3. Devlin, H.B., Plant, J.A. & Griffin, M. (1971) Aftermath of surgery for rectal cancer. *British Medical Journal, iii*, 413–418.
4. MacDonald, L.D. (1982) *Cancer Patients in the Community: Outcomes of Care and Quality of Survival in Rectal Cancer*. Report submitted to the DHSS; June, 1982.

5. Gazzard, B.G. & Dawson, A.M. (1978) Diets and stomas. In *Intestinal Stomas*. Ed. Todd, I. Chap.16, pp.133–149. London: Heinemann.
6. Briggs, M.K., Plant, J.A. & Devlin, H.B. (1977) Labelling the stigmatised: the career of the colostomist. *Annals of Royal College of Surgeons of England, 59*, 248–250.
7. MacDonald, L.D. & Anderson, H.R. (1984) Stigma in patients with rectal cancer: a community study. *Journal of Epidemiology and Community Health, 38*, 284–290.
8. Devlin, H.B. (1981) Digestive diseases and operations. In *Going Home: A Guide for Helping Patients on Leaving Hospital*. Ed. Simpson, J.E.P. & Levill, R. Chap.7, p.78. Churchill Livingstone.

12 Help available for stoma patients

There are various resources available to patients who have a stoma, the aims of which are to enable these individuals to achieve full rehabilitation. This chapter is intended to outline these resources and discuss their specific functions.

THE GENERAL PRACTITIONER

The patient's general practitioner is responsible for his medical care once he leaves hospital. 'His function is to be the main provider of primary and continuing care.'[1] To enable the general practitioner to help his patient he will require prompt clear information from the hospital telling him what has been done and why, how the patient is being managed and what he has been told.[1] The general practitioner will also require information about the appliances and equipment to be used so he can prescribe accurately for the patient; this avoids delay or the patient getting the wrong type or size of appliance. An indication of quantities is also helpful to avoid under or overprescribing.

The general practitioner may see few patients with a stoma compared with those suffering from other diseases (such as hypertension). As stoma patients only form a very small part of his workload, his expertise in this field may be limited. He is, however, in many cases the first person to whom the patient will turn for help and advice when stoma problems arise.[2] The general practitioner will be aware of what help and advice is available locally and can refer the patient to the professional with the relevant expertise. He is also available to the patient to discuss problems and reinforce advice. Hospital personnel tend to change frequently thus the family doctor has the important function of providing continuity.[1] In some cases it is necessary for the patient to obtain a referral from his own doctor for access to other professionals. The general practitioner may also be requested to give information about the patient's condition to other agencies, for example if rehousing is applied for or insurance required.

THE COMMUNITY NURSE

The nurse who visits the patient in his own home after stoma surgery can play a valuable part in his rehabilitation. (See Chapter 11.) Not only does the community nurse deliver the physical nursing care required, but she is also able to form a relationship with the patient and his family. This relationship enables her to develop an understanding of any problems and help seek an appropriate solution. The community nurse can enlist the help and advice of others if required. She may liaise with social services and arrange for practical help in the home if required.

THE SURGEON

The surgeon is a highly skilled specialist who should be consulted to advise on any related surgical problems. Some surgeons see patients who have a stoma on a regular basis as outpatients, while others do not follow them up at all. If complications requiring surgical intervention occur then the patient's general practitioner will refer him to the surgeon. It may be necessary for the surgeon to refashion an unsatisfactory stoma to enable the patient to enjoy as full and normal a life as possible.

THE STOMA CARE NURSE

Many health authorities now employ stoma care nurses. These are Registered General Nurses who have undertaken a specific training course in stoma care. They are clinical specialists and can provide a programme of continuing care and support for patients with a stoma. The role of the stoma care nurse is discussed in the introduction to this book. Most stoma care nurses see patients in hospital and at home, as well as holding clinics where patients have direct access to them and can obtain support and advice.

Stoma care nurses become highly skilled in all aspects of their speciality by merit of training and experience gained in seeing large numbers of stoma patients. Ideally contact with the patient will be made before surgery and she will continue to offer guidance and support for as long as it is required. Working as a member of the team caring for the patient, the stoma care nurse can provide a valuable link between hospital and community. Her expertise can be used as resource for all those professionals who come into contact with stoma patients. Indeed, a primary function is the education of others in the various aspects of stoma care.

The training of stoma care nurses is intended to equip them with skills in counselling and communication as well as knowledge of practical stoma management. They can help patients with most problems relating to stoma surgery or can liaise on the patient's behalf with other professionals who have the relevant expertise.

THE RETAIL PHARMACIST

The retail pharmacist is responsible for dispensing the stoma care equipment prescribed by the patient's doctor. Some pharmacists provide an excellent service for stoma patients (which may include delivery for the frail or elderly) and develop a local reputation. The pharmacist can develop a friendly, trusting relationship with his regular customers for stoma supplies which will enable him to offer advice and information. Some patients may prefer to ask the chemist about a problem rather than trouble the doctor. If the pharmacist knows his customer has a stoma he may be able to caution the patient about the possible effects that any drugs prescribed may have on his bowel function.

In areas where there is no stoma care nurse the pharmacist may be the person to recognize that the patient is using outdated or wrongly sized equipment, he can then query this use and inform the patient of the sources of advice available. Even in areas where there is an efficient stoma care service there will be patients who had their operations years before this facility existed or those who have moved to the area, the so-called 'lost stoma patient'. If the patient agrees, the pharmacist can be instrumental in putting him in touch with the local stoma care nurse.

Patients may request advice from the pharmacist on the use of remedies for problems relating to the stoma and surrounding skin. Self-medication is not usually to be recommended and the pharmacist can encourage and guide the patient to seek professional advice.

APPLIANCE MANUFACTURERS

The appliance manufacturers have played a major role in the research and development of modern stoma appliances. This equipment has enabled those with a stoma to enjoy an improved quality of life.

Most manufacturers can offer information to patients and professionals on the specific use of their products. If more personal enquiries are encountered the patient is usually put in touch with professional help. Some companies have their own nurses who are paid to see patients and advise on their products. The companies that supply stoma care equipment produce useful booklets for patients and professionals. They also support research and education in stoma care and associated diseases.

PATIENT SELF-HELP ASSOCIATIONS

'Ostomy Associations were established in order to provide the new ostomy patient with a contact with a well-rehabilitated ostomist of a number of years standing, who could encourage the new patient to become fully rehabilitated.'[3]

These patient self-help groups are advised by experts from the medical, nursing and legal professions. They are financed by subscription, donation and fund raising. Some receive government help. In Great Britain there are three separate patient self-help associations, and these are described later.

The first patient association was started by a very small group of stoma patients in Philadelphia, USA in the late 1940s. This venture progressed to become the United Ostomy Association of the USA and Canada and now has about 43000 members.[4] In Europe the first patient group to be formed was the Ileostomy Association of Great Britain and Ireland; other countries followed closely. In 1974 the International Ostomy Association was formed and by 1981 there were more than 30 national associations registered.

These self-help groups provide a valuable service for their members, helping to facilitate rehabilitation and teach members to make their lives as normal as possible. It should be part of the stoma care nurse's role to maintain contact with local voluntary organizations who may be able to offer advice and support for individual patients.[5] These groups produce pamphlets which describe their function. Some patients may find it helpful if they are given this written information prior to leaving hospital so that they can make a decision about whether they wish to become involved in such a group.

Patient self-help associations fulfil their function in a variety of ways:

Visiting

A visit from an established stoma patient either in hospital or at home can help the new patient who is undergoing surgery develop more positive attitudes. The visitor can provide living proof that it is possible to look normal after stoma surgery and enjoy a full and active life. Often the patient's fears about social acceptance, recreational activities and other aspects of daily life can be alleviated by discussion with another person who has shared a similar experience. 'The rehabilitated ostomy visitor sets an example of successful rehabilitation and forms a criterion of what can be achieved.'[3] It is beneficial if wherever possible the visitor is matched to the patient according to age, sex, social class and marital status.

The voluntary patient associations will all arrange for a member to visit a new patient on request. These visitors are carefully selected, since it has been found in practice that many individuals are not suitable for this responsible role.[3] They will also have attended a training programme to enable them to function effectively. It is generally agreed that a visiting stoma patient should have lived with his stoma for at least one year, preferably two.[4]

The visitor himself may also benefit from this role as research amongst United Ostomy Association members suggests that visitors' levels of acceptance of their stoma were significantly greater than non-visitors.[6] These differences cannot be directly attributed to the visitor's role, but the findings support the theory that people benefit from helping others. Visiting also provides gratification and an opportunity for social approval.[7]

Welfare services

The patient associations can provide members with practical help, information and advice in dealing with a variety of problems. This may be particularly valuable to the individual stoma patient who encounters prejudice of some kind because he has a stoma. Some of the situations in which the patient associations have been able to exert pressure and overcome prejudice include employment problems, insurance and pension difficulties and the inability to obtain prescribable stoma requisites.

Publications

The patient associations produce well written booklets and information sheets which contain valuable information on a variety of topics. Members are also sent regular journals which contain relevant articles, provide an opportunity for the exchange of views and ideas and carry manufacturer's advertisements to keep the patient abreast of current developments in stoma equipment.

Education and research

Members of the patient associations sometimes participate in research or clinical trials of appliances and equipment. This helps to provide data on which to evaluate the quality of life enjoyed by patients after stoma surgery. National conferences which enable the business of the association to be conducted are often extended to include excellent education programmes which are of benefit to members and interested professionals alike. International meetings are also held.

The patient associations were instrumental in bringing about specialist training for nurses in stoma care. Representatives from these groups often participate in these specialist training courses to inform the nurses of the functions of their association.

The Ileostomy Association (IA)

The Ileostomy Association was founded in 1956. Regular meetings are held (usually biannually) in many major towns and cities throughout Great Britain and Ireland. These meetings usually include displays of equipment by the manufacturing companies.

There is usually a speaker who addresses a topic of interest to ileostomists and a question and answer forum. These gatherings provide members with the opportunity to mix socially and exchange views and ideas. The association also produces a regular journal for its members.

Ileostomy Association of Great Britain and Ireland, Amblehurst House, Chobham, Woking, Surrey. Telephone 099 05 8277

The Urostomy Association (UA)

The Urostomy Association is the newest of the three patient welfare groups, having been established in 1971. It functions along similar lines to the Ileostomy Association.

The Urostomy Association, 'Buckland', Beaumont Park, Danbury, Essex. Telephone 024 541 5294

The Colostomy Welfare Group (CWG)

The Colostomy Welfare Group differs from the other two associations in that it does not hold meetings. The reason for this is that colostomy patients, who are usually in the older age groups, do not always enjoy a good prognosis and it may be distressing for members to identify with others who may have a very short life span. The CWG does, however, offer support to its members in other ways.

Colostomy Welfare Group, 38/39 Eccleston Square, London SW1V 1PB. Telephone 01 828 5175

In some areas stoma patients have formed their own self-help groups which are run to suit the needs of the local population.

FINANCIAL HELP

Some financial help may be available to patients who have a stoma. Although there is no charge for prescriptions other expenses may be incurred such as extra laundry bills particularly if problems arise. Information on the benefits available and how these may be claimed can be obtained from the local Department of Health and Social Security.

The *Disability Rights Handbook*, published by the Disability Alliance ERA, gives information on many aspects of help for the disabled, some of which are pertinent to those with a stoma. Some local authorities have a Welfare Rights Service which can advise individuals on their entitlements and give information on how to go about making claims.

The Disability Alliance ERA, 25 Denmark Street, London WC2H 8NJ. Telephone 01 240 0806

EMPLOYMENT MEDICAL ADVISORY SERVICE (EMAS)

The Employment Medical Advisory Service is an organization of doctors and nurses whose job it is to give advice about occupational health. This free service provides guidance on the placement and return to work of people with health problems. It advises people with health problems about the kind of work that may suit them or that they should avoid.

EMAS does not provide medical treatment but gives specialist advice on the medical aspects of fitness for work, occupational rehabilitation, resettlement and training. The services' occupational health doctors and nurses work closely with disablement resettlement officers of the Manpower Services Commission to help people with health problems find suitable jobs. EMAS also provides medical and nursing services to employment rehabilitation centres which help to prepare people after injury, illness or unemployment for entering or re-entering employment or training. Any doctor may refer a patient who needs an assessment to the medical advisor at the employment rehabilitation centre.

EMAS is part of the Medical Division of the Health and Safety Executive. A leaflet *An Introduction to the Employment Medical Advisory Service* (HSE–5–C200–6/84) is published by the Health and Safety Executive and copies are available from the following address:

The Public Enquiry Point, St Hugh's House, Stanley Precinct, Bootle, Merseyside L20 3QY

DISABLEMENT RESETTLEMENT OFFICER

The disablement resettlement officer is available at the job centre or employment office. He can be contacted without a referral and will explain what employment services are available to those with a disability. He is able to offer a specialized placement and advisory service. There are a number of training schemes and special schemes available which may help the disablement resettlement officer to place people, such as the Job Introduction Scheme.

SEXUAL AND PERSONAL RELATIONSHIPS OF THE DISABLED (SPOD)

SPOD is a charity which became active in 1975 after research indicated that there was a need for specialized workers qualified to give advice to disabled persons with regard to difficulties and problems pertaining to sexual and personal relationships. The aims of the organization are:

1. To stimulate public and professional awareness of sexual needs and difficulties amongst disabled people and of measures that may alleviate their problem in this respect.
2. To provide a centre for the collection and dissemination of information in this field, for disabled people themselves and for those concerned in their welfare.
3. To provide an advisory referral service for disabled clients, therapists, counsellors and educators.
4. To arrange for the training of those working amongst the disabled in the sexual aspects of disability.

While many stoma patients are not disabled they can still make use of this service and benefit from the practical advice and expertise available. SPOD can arrange for personal consultations or may send advice by letter if this is preferable to the client.

The organization also produces advisory leaflets designed to 'provide factual information and advice which may overcome or reduce the sexual problems which are met with by many disabled people'. These advisory leaflets cover several subjects, for example Leaflet 10 *Sex and the Person with an Ostomy* is specifically written for those with a stoma. There are also information sheets available on pertinent topics, and resource lists which recommend reading material relevant to various client groups. All these publications are available by post at a nominal charge.

Sexual and Personal Relationships of the Disabled, 286 Camden Road, London N7 0BJ. Telephone 01 607 8851/2

FAMILY PLANNING ASSOCIATION

The Family Planning Association does not limit its activities to birth control. It also provides advice and counselling for those experiencing sexual difficulties.

THE MARRIAGE GUIDANCE COUNCIL

The Marriage Guidance Council, despite its title, does not just help those experiencing marital disharmony; it provides help for any individual who has a worry about personal relationships, or lack of them. Clients do not have to be married or have a regular relationship. The Council also has sex therapists who are specially trained to provide an individually planned programme of help for couples who have a basically good relationship but are experiencing sexual difficulties. The Marriage Guidance Council has counsellors in most areas and a comprehensive reading list is available.

The National Marriage Guidance Council, Herbert Gray College, Little Church Street, Rugby CV21 3AP. Telephone 0788 73241

REFERENCES

1. Alexander, F.G. (1977) The role of the general practitioner in stoma care. *Practitioner* (July), *219*, 79–84
2. Mitchell, A. (1980) Patients' views on stoma care. *Nursing Mirror*, (3 July), 38–41
3. International Ostomy Association Professional Advisory Committee (1981) Advisory Pamphlet No. 2.
4. Alexander, N.B. (1982) Self-help groups — part I. In *Clinics in Gastroenterology, 11*, 405–414

5. DHSS (1979) *The Provision of Stoma Care.* UK Department of Health Paper HMSO, London
6. Trainor, M.A. (1982) Acceptance of ostomy and the visitor role in a self-help group for ostomy patients. *Nursing Research, 31,* 102–106
7. Trainor, M.A. (1982) Self-help groups — part II. *Clinics in Gastroenterology, 11,* 415–419.

13 The management of enterocutaneous fistula

One of the most exacting challenges nurses meet when looking after surgical patients is encountered in those patients who have developed an enterocutaneous fistula,[1] that is, a connection from a hollow viscus directly to the body surface. This condition is most frequently seen following intestinal anastomosis but may be due to a disease process such as Crohn's disease or to trauma. Once a fistula has formed, intestinal contents can spill out uncontrolled directly onto the patient's skin.

These patients require meticulous and comprehensive care and our efforts to overcome potential problems and achieve a high standard of nursing can be quite exacting. Historically alimentary tract fistulae have been attended by a high mortality and, until comparatively recently, fistulae both traumatic and spontaneous had, in general, a poor prognosis.[2] If the nurse is to be successful when caring for patients with a fistula she must plan her strategy with precision. She may find her ingenuity taxed to the limit in her efforts to overcome the problems encountered in this area of her work.

Fortunately, there have been several discoveries in recent years which have enabled medical and nursing staff to deal more effectively with the many aspects of fistula care. These advances in our knowledge and technology have provided us with some very useful resources which must be exploited to their full potential and carefully planned tactics are necessary if we are to achieve a satisfactory outcome of care.

THE NURSING OBJECTIVES

If the nurse is to be successful in caring for a patient with a fistula she must be clear as to what her objectives are. There are four specific nursing objectives when caring for patients with fistulae.[2]

1. To fit and maintain appliances so that at all times the patient is dry and comfortable.
2. To protect the skin around the fistula from discharge that can cause excoriation and leakage.
3. To ensure all losses are collected and their volume measured to allow deficits to be counteracted.
4. To do everything possible to maintain patient morale. The nurse must also ensure that all prescribed treatment (e.g. drugs, nutritional supplements, etc.) is given accurately and punctually.

A comprehensive nursing assessment of the patient must first be made, which should also include a careful physical assessment of the area surrounding the fistula. We do not have the advantage of choosing a site for a fistula as we do when we predetermine the site of stomas. (See Chapter 9.) The outlet may be anywhere on the abdominal wall or elsewhere on the body surface: in a wound; from a drain site; in a body crease; or near a bony prominence.

The encounter can be all the more arduous since these bodily contours provide ideal channels for leakage to occur. The size and shape of the fistula and its location in relation to other anatomical features must be considered. The nurse must carefully assess the patient's physique and in making this assessment it is helpful to ask the patient to adopt various postures such as sitting, bending and twisting as this changes the body's contours. These changes must be accommodated successfully or leakproof collection of drainage will be compromised. Careful examination of the skin surrounding the fistula may enable the nurse to see possible leakage tracts and focus on these when assembling a drainage system. If there is skin excoriation then urgent treatment may be required, the direction of spread of any excoriation may give us clues as to the sites of previous leakage.

POSSIBLE PROBLEMS WHEN CARING FOR PATIENTS WITH A FISTULA

To plan the patient's care the nurse must be aware of the potential problems she may encounter.

Skin problems

It is crucial that the skin surrounding the fistula is kept dry and healthy.[3] The causes of severe skin damage are related to the quantity and nature of the leakage.[4]

Possible causes

Copious fluid discharge

This may contain a detergent such as bile, which attacks the skin by removing its natural protective film.

Enzymes

These can be a particular problem when dealing with biliary and upper intestinal fistulae. They assault the skin and damage tissues as a result of their digestive capabilities.

Skin excoriation

This will quickly appear if intestinal loss is in contact with the skin. Indiscriminate damage to tissue can have devastating results.

Leakage

Leakage will occur if the collecting appliances are not carefully chosen and applied. This will allow the discharge to contact the skin as well as causing odour and discomfort to the patient. When leakage occurs the nurse will have to change the appliances too frequently, perhaps several times each day, which further compromises painful excoriated skin.

Physiological problems

Sepsis

This used to be a very formidable danger, often capable of defeating all other efforts to cope with a fistula.

Fluid and electrolyte

Imbalance of fluids and electrolytes due to copious losses via the fistula can be readily responsible for the patient's demise.

Malnutrition

Due to the patient's inability to digest and absorb essential nutrients and trace elements malnutrition is capable of undermining the body's ability to defend itself and eventually even to function adequately.

Psychological problems

Low morale

This often results when the effects of one or more of the other problems have taken their toll. Not surprisingly, negative mental attitudes develop — even the most stoical patient will find it difficult to maintain his morale under these circumstances.[3] The patient is often at a low ebb and a psychological attitude of despondency can quickly result, rendering any efforts at further care compromised. It may not only be the patient's morale that is undermined; other members of the caring team may be adversely affected by the slow struggle to overcome these problems and restore the patient to health. Miles Irving comments that the complication of fistula following surgery is an insult to the surgeon's pride.[5]

Odour is often distressing for the patient and others, and the patient's family may also have difficulty maintaining a positive attitude in the face of prolonged illness in their loved one.

Management problems

Inappropriate surgery

To close the fistula inappropriate surgery may be attempted. This is usually thought to be inadvisable,[2] since it may add little to the cause and can result in further problems manifesting.

It looks a very gloomy picture when we view these problems. Little imagination is need to understand how, without the resources more recently available, few patients with fistula survived.

RESOURCES AVAILABLE TO THE NURSE

To enable her to plan the patient's care the nurse must be aware of what resources are at her disposal to meet the patient's individual needs.

Protecting the skin

Skin barriers

Barriers are now available which can be used to protect the skin from leakage and enzyme attack. They will adhere to moist excoriated skin and form a protective layer that can remain effective for several days even in the presence of copious losses containing intestinal enzymes.   `

Modern stoma care appliances

These can be used effectively to contain effluent so that excoriation does not occur and the patient is spared the discomfort of leakage. However, many patients equate wearing such an appliance with having a stoma. It is therefore, essential to reassure the patient that this is not the case, provided that this is true. Details of suitable products are discussed in Chapter 4.

Overcoming physiological problems

Antibiotics

It is now possible to overcome most sepsis provided these modern powerful agents are given systematically and used discriminately.

Intravenous fluids

These can replace fluids lost from the body via the fistula. Provided the nursing team can be relied upon to make accurate recordings on input and output charts, fluid balance can be achieved.

Electrolyte replacement

Following biochemical analysis of blood and fistula effluent, electrolyte replacement will facilitate the body's chemical processes continuing unimpaired.

Intensive nutritional support

This has been demonstrated to close the majority of enterocutaneous fistulae,[6] rendering surgery unnecessary. New technology in the nutritional field now makes it possible to nourish the patient adequately by either supplementing or replacing the diet with high protein, low residue feeds. There are several ready-to-use products available which can be taken orally or can be instilled via a fine-bore nasogastric tube into the gastrointestinal tract. These provide all the nutrients, vitamins and trace elements essential for a balanced diet. Some surgeons favour the nutrients being in a predigested form as an elemental diet.[3]

In cases where a fistula is very high in the tract a feeding enterostomy may be indicated. If the gut is functional and the patient can absorb nutrients this should be the route of choice for feeding. If it is not suitable to feed the patient via this route then total nourishment can be achieved via the parenteral route. The old adage 'feed the fistula' holds much truth as tissue repair and healing will be compromised in a malnourished patient.

Dealing with psychological problems

It is essential that all those involved in the patient's care join forces to elevate and maintain the patient's morale at as high a level as possible. Frequent consultation between all the team members is essential as the patient's condition changes rapidly.[1] Any measure to lessen anxiety and promote positive attitudes are worth while. The patient and his family will be in need of explanation and support throughout this often lengthy process of healing. Sensitive counselling is essential, thus the nurse must have empathy with the patient and attempt to build an understanding relationship to facilitate this helping process. Nursing care plans must be flexible and evaluated regularly so that they can be adapted to meet the patient's changing needs.[1]

The patient's family should be encouraged to visit regularly and help to sustain his psychological well-being. Any form of diversional therapy that can catch the patient's interest is worth pursuing, be it jigsaws or basket making. Attention should also be directed to the patient's general appearance; the nurse must ensure that he has shaved, is in clean pyjamas and his hair is combed to help maintain his self-respect. Appliance covers should be used to help prevent sweating and to hide the contents of the bags from view. Most manufacturers have functional covers available but much more attractive disguises can be home-made.

The fight against declining morale can be an exacting encounter. Both psychology and ingenuity must be pressed into service together with any other tactics to avoid defeat.

Management considerations

To enable its members to function efficiently the care team may also need psychological support, particularly the nursing staff who are with the patient for extended periods of time. With the advent of patient allocation and the nursing process the nurse now gets much closer to the patient emotionally. Ward meetings and discussion with other team members will help the nurse to cope with this type of stress.[7] Medical staff may likewise need support from their peer group, as it is essential that all team members remain astute and well motivated.

Well-planned surgery

Once some of these other problems have been overcome the surgeon may consider it appropriate to operate, possibly to deal with the damaged bowel and create a diverting stoma, such as a loop ileostomy proximal to the fistula.[2]

To enable her to gain the maximum benefit from these resources the nurse must use them appropriately. The nursing care plan must be drawn up with considerable thought and precision, being evaluated and modified when indicated.

STRATEGY FOR CARING FOR A PATIENT WITH A FISTULA

(A more detailed description of the products used appears in Chapter 4.)

1. The nurse must be in possession of all the relevant information about the patient from her nursing assessment.
2. All equipment must be assembled before commencing the dressing. It is often necessary to enlist the help of a second nurse to act as assistant.
3. The skin should be cleansed with an anionic solution such as cetrimide. If there is a high output from the fistula a suction line operated continuously by an assistant will remove any discharge and keep the field dry until the dressing is complete. If no assistant is available it may be possible to control the output either by gently syringing the outlet or by putting a balloon catheter into the fistula and inflating the balloon to act as a stopper for a short time.
4. The surrounding skin must be gently shaved, taking care not to damage the skin further; this will aid adhesion and prevent undue discomfort when dressings are changed.
5. The fistula should be gently explored to assess its size and determine if it has one or more openings.
6. To promote good leakproof adhesion of a collecting appliance the skin must be levelled and rendered flat. This can be achieved by applying a filler paste into each crevice or delve, and building up layers until a flat surface is achieved. Many of these filler pastes contain alcohol and therefore cause a transient stinging when applied to damaged skin. A sprinkling of barrier powder can help alleviate this.
7. Once the skin surface is level a flat barrier wafer can be applied to protect the skin from contact with effluent. If a level surface has not been achieved then seepage can occur beneath the barrier wafer, lifting it from the skin. To facilitate accurate fitting of the barrier wafer a template should be made from thin card. This is most easily achieved by placing an acetate sheet over the area and tracing the shape with a marking pen. This pattern can then be transferred to the card and an exact template cut out. The barrier wafer should be placed in position and gently massaged onto the skin, allowing the heat from the hands to

enhance adhesion. Warm air from a hair-drier can be very useful to increase the malleability and adhesion of the barrier wafer. If the immediate area is recessed a series of radial cuts can be made to enable the wafer to be pressed into its margins, and gaps may then be filled with paste. It is important not to allow the wafer to overlap the fistula opening, lest fluid tracks beneath. Time spent in accurate cutting and placement of the wafer is well rewarded. In summary, the aim is to apply a protective barrier wafer to cover all the skin up to the very margins of the fistula opening. Once this has been achieved a suitable appliance can be fitted.

8. There is a wide variety of products available and most ileostomy appliances can prove suitable. The appliance must be drainable and odourproof; transparent plastic provides ease of observation. Some two-piece appliances incorporate a flange made from barrier wafer which can be cut and fitted as previously described and then the appliance attached.

9. If a one-piece appliance is to be used a gasket size slightly larger than the fistula opening is most suitable, provided the surrounding skin is protected with a barrier wafer.

In cases where there is a very high fluid output a urostomy appliance attached to a night drainage bag may prove most suitable to avoid the bag requiring too frequent emptying or becoming detached due to excess weight.

Provided these steps are followed it is quite possible to assemble a collecting appliance that will remain secure for several days. Once a leakproof system of collection has been achieved the patient should be able to move around and be free from the discomfort and embarrassment of leakage. The skin is protected from the effluent and accurate measuring and analysis of the output is possible.

MULTIPLE FISTULAE

The problems encountered when coping with multiple fistulae can be somewhat more complicated. It is desirable where possible to collect the output from each fistula individually. In order to achieve this the whole area must be protected as previously described with a barrier wafer. This may entail using one very large wafer or joining several smaller ones, filling any defects around joins with paste. Provided the outlets do not lie too close to each other, several small appliances can then be applied, one over each discharging site. A mouldable flat drainable appliance with adhesive only is often useful, the adhesives can overlap each other allowing the bags to be applied very close together.[2]

1. If the drainage holes lie deep in a wound they can be separated by building a 'dam' made from paste and skin barrier wafer. (See Figs 44 and 45.) The edges of the wound are coated with protective powder then a dam is built by putting a layer of filler paste, topped by a flattened roll of

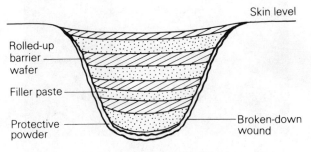

Fig. 44. *Cross-section of a 'dam'.*

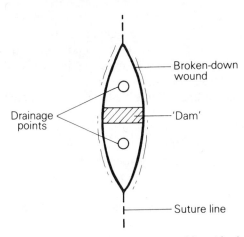

Fig. 45. *Two leakage points separated by a 'dam'.*

skin barrier wafer, followed by a further layer of paste, then barrier wafer, etc., until the dam reaches skin level; two separate appliances can then be applied once the surrounding area is protected by a barrier wafer.[8]

2. If there are several outlets close together then one large collecting appliance may be the most practical solution. Some larger appliances incorporate a protective wafer which may be cut using a template as described. Others which incorporate an adhesive area only should be fitted onto a separate barrier wafer. (See Fig. 46.)

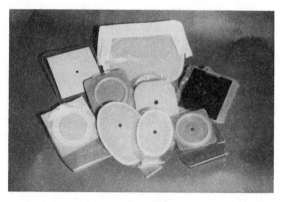

Fig. 46. *A selection of large appliances suitable for use with multiple fistulae.*

3. Suction drainage of a fistula is rarely indicated but it may be essential in the early management of high output fistulae from the depth of an irregular wound. This will control the effluent until a track has formed enabling an appliance to be fitted.[9] In these cases once the area is cleansed and kept dry with a suction line, a large balloon catheter may be inserted into the outlet and the surrounding canyon filled with silastic foam. This forms a plug which may be removed and cleaned. The surrounding skin can be protected with a barrier wafer and the plug held in position by a stoma belt and a ring. The catheter can then be attached to low pressure suction and any seepage will be absorbed by the foam plug.

4. If further support or adhesion is required for the dressing there are a variety of tapes, belts and seals available.

5. Flatus passing from the fistula may cause the appliance to

distend. In this case one or more charcoal flatus filters can be fitted to provide an escape route for deodorized flatus.

6. Odour can be a problem, particularly in the presence of bacteria. This is distressing to the patient. Hopefully, if a leakproof appliance is fitted odour should only be apparent when bags are emptied or changed. Good ventilation is essential but must be discreet. An air freshener should be used and products are available to go inside the appliance which disguise or absorb odour.

Patients with a fistula rely on team care; we must rely on the medical staff to prescribe adequate and appropriate regimes for fluid and electrolyte replacement, antibiotic therapy and, in conjunction with the dietician, intensive nutritional support. It is, of course, a nursing responsibility to ensure these regimens are accurately and effectively administered and that the appropriate data for their prescription is available.

All fistulae require exacting management and, fortunately, we are now much better equipped to do battle with a greater chance of success in overcoming the previously poor prognosis for patients with enterocutaneous fistulae. It is a demanding but I feel a very rewarding fight.

REFERENCES

1. Alexander-Williams, J., & Irving, M. (1982) *Intestinal Fistula*, Chap. 5, p.84. Bristol: J. Wright & Son.
2. Devlin, H.B. & Elcoat, C.E. (1983) Alimentary tract fistula: stomatherapy techniques of management. *World Journal of Surgery, 7,*
3. Bentley, R.J. (1976) Intestinal fistula. *Nursing Times*, 2 December. 1879–1880.
4. Winkler, R. & Pfeiffer, M. (1977) Treatment of skin lesions caused by fistulae arising from breakdown of surgical sutures. *Therapie der Gegenwart, 6*, June No.6. 2–7.
5. Irving, M. (1977) Local and surgical management of entero-cutaneous fistulae. *British Journal of Surgery, 64*, 690–694.
6. MacFadyan, B.V., Dudrick, S.J. & Ruberg, R.L. (1973) Management of gastrointestinal fistulae with parenteral hyperalimentation. *Surgery, 74*, 100–105.
7. Dowd, D. & Martin, T. (1984) Oasis on mondays. *Nursing Times*, 17 October, 50–51.
8. Gross, E.R. & Irving, M. (1977) Skin protection around entero-cutaneous fistula. *British Journal of Surgery, 64*, 690.
9. Alexander-Williams, J. & Irving, M. (1982) *Intestinal Fistula*, Chap.4, p.77. Bristol: J. Wright & Son.

14 Complications of stomas

Possible complications faced by patients who have a stoma come into three categories:

- Physiological complications.
- Psychological complications.
- Physical complications.

The possible physiological and psychological problems are discussed elsewhere in this book. (See Chapters 1 and 5.) However, the physical problems, if they occur, can be equally distressing. Some complications will require further surgery while others can be treated with medication and altered techniques in caring for the stoma. This chapter discusses those complications together with the conditions involving the peristomal skin, which may give rise to problems in stoma management.

Abnormal bowel function, such as constipation and diarrhoea, can affect any patient but some particular considerations are necessary when they occur in a patient with a faecal stoma, and these are also highlighted.

COMPLICATIONS WHICH MAY REQUIRE SURGERY

The nurse should report any suspected complications as soon as possible to the doctor in charge of the case so that he can give a medical opinion.

Prolapse

This is a condition in which a length of bowel prolapses out onto the exterior of the abdomen. It is most commonly seen in transverse loop colostomies (see Fig. 47); one study in children revealed this complication in 12% of cases,[1] and others suggest a 20% incidence.[2] Most usually the distal portion of bowel prolapses but the condition can also involve the proximal opening or both openings.[3]

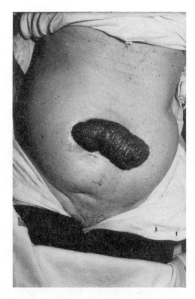

Fig. 47. *A prolapsed transverse colostomy.*

Possible problems

1. The stoma may be prone to trauma due to friction of the appliance against the mucosa.
2. The patient may have difficulty in fitting an appliance, particularly in the case of a large prolapse.
3. The protruding bowel may become oedematous or even necrosed if the appliance is constricting.
4. Intestinal obstruction may occur if the proximal bowel has prolapsed and becomes kinked.
5. The patient often experiences psychological problems as the protruding bowel is unsightly and can be detectable under clothing.

Nursing action

1. A careful explanation should be given to the patient as to what has taken place since he will naturally be alarmed by the sudden increase in the size of his stoma. He will need a lot of psychological support to help him cope. It is essential to give

reassurance that the condition is not serious despite its appearance and that it can be surgically repaired.

2. The patient may need to be fitted with a larger appliance to accommodate the protruding bowel, thus avoiding any pressure or trauma. Vaseline gauze wrapped around the bowel may eliminate friction from the appliance. It is essential to select an appliance with a large enough opening to avoid any constriction in the blood supply to the bowel.

3. Careful instruction will be needed to teach the patient how to fit the larger appliance and cope with the enlarged stoma physically.

4. The patient should be advised to report any change in bowel colour, which may indicate ischaemia or abdominal colic, and any change in stomal function, which may indicate intestinal obstruction.

Treatment

In some cases it is possible to manually reduce the prolapse, particularly if the patient is lying flat. If the stoma is temporary then the prolapse can be dealt with when the stoma is closed. If closure of the colostomy is contraindicated then it may be necessary to divide the loop colostomy, establishing a single opening proximal colostomy and close the distal loop returning it to the abdomen.[3]

Ischaemia

This condition may compromise the stoma as a result of an impaired blood supply. The stoma will appear a dusky purple initially and black when truly necrotic. Necrosis may be due to the establishment of an inadequate blood supply to the bowel when the stoma is formed. However, it can occur due to constriction of the stoma by an appliance that is too small or pressure from bed covers or tightly fitting clothing.

Possible problems

1. Severe ischaemia will render the stoma inviable; it will become gangrenous and will eventually slough off.

2. Due to lack of sensation in the stoma, ischaemia can take place without the patient being aware of it.
3. The appearance and odour of the necrotic stoma can be psychologically traumatic to the patient.

Nursing action

1. Close observation of the stoma during the postoperative period is essential. A clear plastic appliance should be fitted and any change in colour of the mucosa reported to the doctor in charge of the case.
2. The appliance fitted in the immediate postoperative period should be slightly larger than the stoma to allow for any possible swelling avoiding constriction. If a methyl cellulose wafer is used then a series of radial cuts should be made around the opening to facilitate flexibility.
3. If necrosis occurs, the patient will need psychological support and reassurance about the condition. A full explanation of the condition and proposed treatment should be given.
4. The patient should be cautioned about wearing tight constricting clothing over the stoma.

Treatment

In many cases the area of necrosis is confined to the mucosa, the central area being pink in colour. In this situation the necrotic tissue will often slough off leaving a healthy stoma. In cases where the stoma is not viable further surgery is required. It may be possible to draw out more bowel without opening the abdomen but if the gangrene extends too deeply, a laparotomy will be required to excise the affected tissue and reconstruct the stoma.

Stenosis

This is a condition in which the outlet of the stoma becomes narrowed. It can become so severe that the stoma becomes almost closed. Stenosis may be due to scar tissue, inappropriate technique when the stoma is fashioned or severe infection around the stoma resulting in a separation of the bowel and skin. (See Fig. 48.)

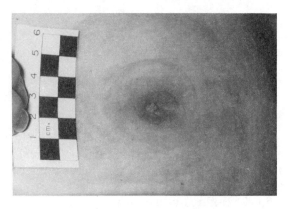

Fig. 48. *Stenosis of a colostomy.*

Possible problems

1. Pain when passing a formed motion via the stoma.
2. Abdominal cramps.
3. Intestinal obstruction.

Treatment

If the stenosis is not too severe, regular digital dilatation may help. However, this must be done with care or more scarring due to tearing of tissues may result. Stool softeners may also be helpful in ensuring that the patient does not become constipated resulting in a hard stool which he is unable to pass. If the stenosis is severe then surgical intervention is necessary. This may be a local plastic correction or the stoma may need to be refashioned in an alternative site.

Retraction

This is a recession of the stoma usually due to the bowel being under tension. It may be caused by too little bowel being mobilized when the stoma is fashioned, inadequate fixing or postoperative weight gain. Removal of the support bridge in a loop stoma can also result in retraction. (See Fig. 49.)

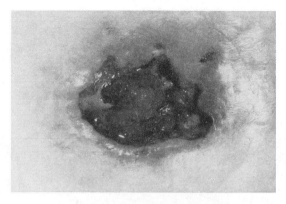

Fig. 49. *A retracted ileostomy.*

Possible problems

1. The stoma may appear satisfactory when the patient is standing but retract when he lies flat. This can result in leakage of effluent under the appliance when the patient is prone, usually at night.
2. Difficulty in fitting and maintaining a secure, leakproof appliance. This can result in skin excoriation.
3. Psychological problems resulting from leakage.

Treatment

In less severe cases the patient may benefit from wearing an appliance with a rigid flange and a belt worn securely to depress the surrounding skin, thus forcing the stoma to protrude. However, it is of paramount importance that no pressure is put onto the stoma itself. A reduction in the patient's weight may be advantageous, particularly if there has been an increase since surgery. In more severe cases surgical refashioning is required.

Herniation

Herniation around the colostomy is frequently seen in iliac 'end' colostomies. About 20–25% of cases develop peristomal herniae.[2] It is less common in ileostomy patients. The degree of herniation can vary from a slight bulge when the patient coughs to a large

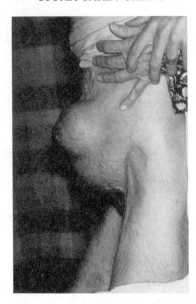

Fig. 50. *A paracolostomy hernia.*

unsightly hernia with the stoma at its apex or, perhaps worse, beneath the hernia bulge. The condition is usually more prevalent in the older age group due to diminished muscle tone. (See Fig. 50.)

Possible problems

1. The shape of the hernia may make fitting an appliance more difficult; this problem is compounded if the stoma is hidden from the patient's view by the hernia.
2. Large hernias can cause the patient considerable embarrassment resulting in psychological problems.
3. Intestinal obstruction can occur, due to kinking or twisting of bowel within the hernia.
4. Irrigation of the stoma is much more difficult.

Nursing action

1. The nurse must reassure the patient about the hernia and its cause. Many patients fear that the 'lump' is a recurrence of the cancer they have had excised.

2. The patient may need to select an alternative more flexible appliance that will still fit snugly despite the stoma not now being on a planar surface. The patient may also need to learn a revised technique for fitting his appliance if his stoma is hidden by the hernia, e.g. by using a shaving mirror to ensure accurate placement.
3. The patient should be made aware of the signs and symptoms of intestinal obstruction and asked to report any change in his stoma function.
4. If the patient has been previously managing his colostomy by irrigation this may now be contraindicated and the nurse may need to help the patient select a suitable appliance.

Treatment

In mild cases no treatment at all may be advised. Sometimes the patient may feel more comfortable wearing an elastic support belt with the appropriate opening for the stoma. In more severe cases surgery to resite the stoma may be indicated but there is a risk of herniation at the new site. It may be possible in some cases to repair the hernia leaving the stoma site unchanged.

Fistula

A fistula can occur at the base of the stomal spout in the case of ileostomy and ileal conduit. This will allow effluent to seep from the lumen of the stoma onto the abdomen at skin level. If the fistula occurs in the postoperative period it is most commonly due to a stitch being passed through the full thickness of the bowel.[3] If the fistula occurs at a later stage it may be due to pressure from an ill-fitting or poorly applied appliance.[4,5] Another possible cause is Crohn's disease.[5]

Possible problems

1. Inability to fit a secure leakproof appliance.
2. Skin excoriation due to leakage as the effluent is exuded at skin level it will often seep beneath the collecting appliance.

Nursing action

1. The patient will need an explanation of why the leakage is occurring and the plan of treatment.
2. It may be possible for the nurse to develop a system for containing the effluent as with other enterocutaneous fistulae. (See Chapter 13.)
3. It is essential to teach the patient careful measuring of the stoma to ensure the correct size of appliance is selected. The patient must also be aware of the importance of following a technique resulting in accurate fitting.

Treatment

In some cases the fistula may close if the pressure is removed and the patient's general condition is good. However, it is frequently necessary for surgical revision of the stoma.

Avulsion

This is a condition where the spout of the ileostomy is torn off due to trauma, most usually caused by a seat belt in a road traffic accident.[6]

Treatment

Surgery is required to construct a new ileostomy as soon as possible.

Cancer colonization of the stoma

A recurrence of carcinoma around the stoma can occur if inadequate clearance has been achieved when the cancer is excised or from spread through the lymphatics. Another cause may be peritoneal deposits giving rise to a growth near the stoma. Cancer colonization (Fig. 51) is rare in ileostomies as they are rarely constructed in malignant disease. In the case of ilial conduits the malignancy in the bladder is divorced from the ileum involved in the stoma.

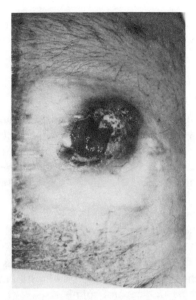

Fig. 51. *Cancer colonization around a colostomy.*

Possible problems

1. The patient may encounter great problems in coping with this complication psychologically.
2. The carcinoma may cause stenosis and eventually obstruction of the stoma.
3. Problems may be encountered in fitting an appliance.

Nursing action

1. The patient will need sensitive psychological support and counselling.
2. The nurse may need to help the patient select an appliance that will accommodate the stoma and growth.
3. The patient should be told the signs of obstruction and asked to report any change in his stomal function.

Treatment

The treatment will be governed primarily by the patient's general condition and prognosis. In some cases surgical intervention may be appropriate. Stool softeners may be useful if the colostomy outlet becomes too narrow to excrete a formed motion.

Bleeding

Bleeding from a stoma may be due to a variety of causes. Minor bleeding from the surface of the stoma during an appliance change may be due to overenthusiastic cleansing and can be likened to the gums bleeding when the teeth are scrubbed. Another cause of bleeding from the surface of the stoma is a granuloma, which is usually a result of repeated trauma, such as from the rigid flange of an appliance.[5]

Bleeding from the lumen of the stoma is potentially more serious; it may be due to varices caused by portal hypertension in the case of liver cirrhosis or hepatic metastases. A recurrence of colonic carcinoma can also result in bleeding as well as stomal dysfunction. Other disease of the gastrointestinal tract may result in bleeding, such as an ulcer in Crohn's disease eroding a vessel or peptic ulceration.

Treatment

All bleeding from the lumen of a stoma warrants careful investigation so that a diagnosis can be made. The treatment will vary depending upon the cause of the haemorrhage; it may include surgery.

If varices of the stoma are causing bleeding an injection of phenol or pressure may be helpful. In the case of a bleeding granuloma pressure with cotton gauze will usually stem the flow. Cautery with a silver nitrate stick will usually resolve the problem provided the source of the pressure is discovered and eliminated. If surface bleeding is thought to be due to overenthusiastic cleaning then correcting the patient's technique is all that is required.

Ileostomy obstruction

Obstruction of an ileostomy may be due to food volvulus, bands of adhesions, paraileostomy hernia, stenosis or recurrence of a disease such as Crohn's disease resulting in stricture formation.

The ileostomy appears tense and oedematous and may discharge fluid effluent prior to complete cessation of function. The patient usually experiences severe abdominal colic, distension, vomiting and bowel sounds are increased and high pitched. The patient can become very ill due to fluid and electrolyte balance disorders which can quickly ensue. Increased osmolarity of gut contents causes water to pass into the gut, resulting in eventual decrease in blood volume.[7] This can be a very serious complication and urgent medical intervention is indicated.

Treatment

The patient will often require intravenous infusion of fluid and nasogastric aspiration to counteract the effect of the obstruction. The cause of the obstruction should be ascertained and an erect and supine abdominal X-ray is usually ordered. If a volvulus is suspected this may clear spontaneously, particularly if the patient is given sedation to ease the pain and help relax the gut.

Irrigation of the ileostomy using a *soft fine rubber catheter* and warm sterile saline solution may bring relief, or the blockage may be partially overcome leaving the intestine to complete the task.[8] In cases where the obstruction persists emergency surgery is indicated to elicit and correct the cause.

Foods which are high in cellulose and difficult to digest can cause an obstruction, e.g. cauliflower, peanuts, coconut and beans/sprouts. It is therefore essential that patients with ileostomies have adequate dietary advice. (See Chapter 16.)

SKIN COMPLICATIONS

Excoriation

This is caused when faeces or urine are allowed to come into contact with the skin. The effect is similar to leaving a child in a soiled napkin—the skin becomes sore. This problem is compounded in the case of an ileostomy patient where the effluent may be strongly alkaline and contain the proteolytic enzymes of digestion.

Assessment

1. The nurse should take an accurate history from the patient and elicit the details regarding the excoriation:
   - Has the patient gained or lost weight?
   - Has the size or shape of the stoma altered?
   - Has the effluent changed in nature?
   - Has any leakage occurred onto the skin outside the appliance?
   - Does the leakage occur during any particular activity?

2. An examination of the area around the stoma may indicate the cause of excoriation. If there are any particular tracks visible where excoriation has occurred this may indicate a skin crease along which effluent has been in contact with the skin. The patient should be asked to adopt various positions as these movements may reveal creases that are not apparent when the patient is lying flat.
   The size of the stoma should also be checked since if it retracts when the patient is supine this can cause faeces to exude at skin level and track beneath the adhesive surface of the appliance. A fistula at the base of the stoma can also allow this to occur.

3. The size of the gasket or opening cut into the appliance should be closely compared to the size and shape of the stoma. There should be no more than 3 mm of peristomal skin exposed. A ring of excoriation around the base of the stoma is often a sign that the wrong size of appliance is being used.

4. Examination of a used appliance may reveal the tracks where leakage has occurred.

5. It is helpful to ask the patient to carry out an appliance change while the nurse observes. This should be done in the position that the patient usually adopts to change his bag and he should not alter his technique in any way. Observation may reveal a fault in the method of application.

6. The cleansing and drying of the skin should also be questioned and the nurse should elicit if any topical applications are being used on the peristomal skin since this may compromise adhesion of the appliance. When the appliance is in place the nurse should check if it is adhering securely.

Possible problems

1. Wrongly sited stoma that allows leakage to occur via a skin crease or due to a protruding bony prominence.[5] (See Chapter 9.)
2. Too short a spout being achieved when the stoma is fashioned. This is particularly important in the case of ileostomy and urinary stomas where the effluent is fluid. Ideally the stoma should be approximately 2.5 cm in length.[5]
3. If the wrong type of appliance is being used or the appliance is incorrectly fitted this can allow leakage to occur or the unprotected skin to become excoriated. The appliance should fit snugly around the stoma protecting all the peristomal skin but not constricting the stoma in any way.[9] It may be necessary to use a particularly flexible appliance in cases where the stoma is inappropriately placed.

Nursing action

Using the information gathered the nurse should try to elicit what she thinks is the problem in each individual case. She can then plan the care the patient will require to achieve healthy peristomal skin.

Problem: wrong type or size of appliance. The nurse should help the patient to select an appliance that will meet his individual needs. If the appliance being used was the wrong size then this should be rectified after careful measuring. The patient should be

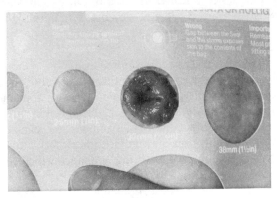

Fig. 52. *Measuring a stoma.*

taught to measure his stoma regularly and check that the opening in his appliance is the correct size. This is particularly important in the postoperative periods when the stoma size often changes substantially due to decreasing oedema in the tissue. (See Fig. 52.)

Problem: leakage due to patient's physique. If leakage occurs because the appliance is unable to bond securely due to the patient's physique then an alternative appliance should be selected. If the stoma is inappropriately positioned or the patient has gained or lost weight the area onto which the appliance fits may not be flat. A very flexible appliance with no rigid flange or gasket is often the most successful in adhering to the body's contours and eliminating leakage.

Problem: leakage due to skin creases. Skin creases form ideal channels along which effluent can pass, causing leakage and excoriation. These creases may not be apparent when the patient is standing or lying flat but when he bends, twists or crouches the crease may appear. These movements must be accommodated if the patient is to lead a full and active life. The nurse should teach the patient to fill in these creases using a proprietary filling paste before the appliance is fitted. It may be helpful to teach the patient to pull his abdominal skin taught prior to fitting his appliance so that no creases are secured beneath the adhesive.

Problem: incorrect fitting technique. If the nurse can elicit faults when watching the patient change his appliance then these should be corrected diplomatically. It is important to explain to the patient what the mistake is and why his technique for fitting the appliance allows leakage to occur.

Problem: excoriated skin/compromised adhesion. Once the skin becomes excoriated, it is often painful, broken and 'weeping'. In this situation it is impossible to fit some types of appliance as the adhesive will not adhere to the weeping broken skin. In such cases it is essential to protect the skin from further damage due to contact with effluent, thus allowing it to heal. A methyl cellulose skin wafer can be fitted beneath the appliance which will protect the skin and enable healing to occur. These skin wafers will adhere even to moist skin and can absorb small amounts of exudate. Some two-piece appliances incorporate such a wafer and these may prove very suitable in some cases. However, if they feature a rigid flange, it may preclude their use with some patients.

The use of a drainable appliance that can remain *in situ* for two to three days is often advantageous in allowing the skin to heal without frequently disturbing the appliance. When the skin is intact the patient can resume use of a closed pouch if suitable.

Problem: not identified. There are some cases when it is not possible to find a definite cause for the leakage. It may prove helpful to assist the patient in selecting an alternative appliance to try. It is essential to educate patients with a stoma in the care of the peristomal skin and the importance of following a careful technique to avoid damage to the skin.

It is worth while to note that some patients may complain of leakage despite every effort to overcome the problem. If no problem can be identified it may be that this is the patient's way of asking for help; an excuse to see the nurse. This should be particularly considered if no excoriation of the skin is apparent. In such cases careful questioning may reveal the true problem and counselling may then be the most appropriate action.

Irritation

Skin irritation occurs when an irritant substance is absorbed into the lower living layers of the skin.

Assessment

1. The nurse should take an accurate history from the patient and elicit details of the irritation.
2. An examination of the area around the stoma will reveal any breaks in the peristomal skin and the area of irritation can also be defined.
3. The nurse should identify the type of appliance being used and ascertain any features that may be relevant, e.g. occlusive adhesive which will not allow the skin to 'breathe'.
4. Careful questioning about skin care and the products used may reveal that the patient is applying a highly irritant substance to the skin or is undermining the skin's defences.

Possible problems

1. Damage to the outer horny layers of skin, allowing irritant substances to be absorbed.
2. The topical application of strongly irritant substances to the peristomal skin.
3. Use of an occlusive substance on the skin causing increased temperature and humidity which will, in turn, increase the rate of absorption of irritant substance.

Nursing action

Problem: damaged protective outer skin layer. The cause of such damage should be identified and eliminated. The outer layer of skin should then be protected to allow it to heal; a methyl cellulose wafer applied to the peristomal skin may help in allowing the skin the remain undisturbed for several days thus enhancing healing.

If a topical application is required to soothe and promote healing this should be non-greasy so as not to compromise adhesion of the appliance. Use of barrier cream or gel may help reduce the absorption of irritant substances.

Problem: topical application of irritant substance. If the nurse can identify an irritant substance that the patient is using then this should be eliminated. Perfume or talcum powder being trapped beneath the adhesive of the appliance and subsequently absorbed is a common cause of irritation. The use of soap around the stoma should also be avoided since this removes the natural surface lipids from the skin making it more vulnerable. Strong or scented soaps may prove to be irritant themselves. Plain water is usually adequate to cleanse the skin.

It is important to impress on the patient that he should not apply anything irritant to the skin and fully explain the reason why.

Problem: occlusive appliance. If the patient is using an appliance that features an occlusive adhesive the nurse should explain the possible action in raising the temperature and increasing sweating. She should then assist the patient in selecting an alternative but suitable modern appliance with an adhesive that allows skin function to continue unimpaired in normal conditions.

Physical damage

Physical damage occurs when the outer skin cells are constantly being removed from the surface, thus exposing the lower layers of skin. This can usually be identified since the area of damage will correspond to the area of the adhesive on the appliance.

Assessment

1. The nurse should take a careful account of how frequently the patient changes his appliance.
2. Information should be obtained about the pattern of stomal action and the consistency of the motions.
3. The nurse should ascertain what prompts the patient to decide that he needs to change his appliance.
4. Identification of the type of appliance being used will reveal whether it incorporates an aggressive adhesive.
5. Examination of the peristomal skin will reveal the area of damage; this may correspond to the total area of adhesion or perhaps just to the area not protected by a ring or washer. The condition of the abdominal skin generally should also be noted.

Possible problems

1. Too frequent changing of the appliance. Each time the adhesive is removed from the skin an outer layer of cells will also be removed.
2. The adhesive of the appliance being too aggressive and removing several outer layers of cells when it is changed.
3. The abdominal skin is very tender and easily damaged, and is therefore very susceptible to physical damage.

Nursing action

Problem: too frequent changing of appliance. If the appliance is being changed too frequently then the nurse should consider what the patient gives as his reason for deciding to change the bag.

It may be that the patient has a fluid or semi-fluid stool but uses a closed appliance. In this case a drainable bag that remains in situ on the skin but can be emptied as frequently as necessary is more suitable. The nurse should help the patient select a suitable drainable appliance. Some patients may feel that it is necessary to change the appliance each time the stoma acts in an endeavour to feel 'clean'. In this situation counselling is required to explore why the patient should feel this need for frequent changing and to elicit any other problems, e.g. leakage or odour.

Education is then required to ensure that the patient develops an acceptable routine and appreciates the problems that arise from frequent changing. If the problem persists the patient may benefit from using a two-piece appliance so that the skin remains undisturbed when the bag is changed.

Problem: excessively strong adhesive. Many modern stoma care appliances feature an acrylic adhesive which is light and less likely to damage the skin tissues when removed. The patient may benefit from changing to such an appliance which has a gentle adhesive.

Problem: vulnerable abdominal skin. If the patient's abdominal skin is frail it should be protected from damage as much as possible. A two-piece appliance is often the most suitable as the flange is only removed from the skin about twice weekly. Alternatively, an application of a protective film prior to each appliance change may prove beneficial.

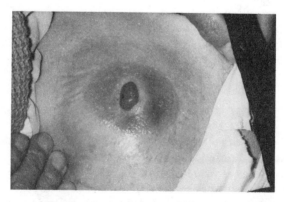

Fig. 53. *Allergic reaction to a skin protective.*

Sensitivity/allergy

The skin may be sensitive to certain substances, this is the result of exposure to a particular allergen and the formation of antibodies. Re-exposure results in lymphocytes being formed which cause a skin reaction. (See Fig. 53.)

Assessment

1. A history of the allergic reaction should be sought and attempts made to discover if its occurrence coincided with any alteration in skin care or use of products.
2. Examination of the peristomal skin will reveal the area of the reaction. The culprit may be immediately identified if it is only one particular area that is affected, e.g. if the area in contact with the protective washer shows a reaction but the area under the adhesive is healthy.
3. The nurse should elicit from the patient details of any substance to which he has been allergic in the past.

Possible problems

The skin is sensitized to a certain substance, this could be:

1. The adhesive of the appliance.
2. The skin protective of the appliance.
3. Plastic.
4. Products used on skin, e.g. barrier cream.

Nursing action

The substance causing the allergy must be identified and eliminated. If identification is obvious then a change to an alternative appliance with a different type of adhesive, flange or wafer may be successful. If the allergen cannot be readily identified then patch testing may be required. This involves fixing small pieces of the suspect substance to another area of skin (such as the underside of the arm) and eliciting if a reaction occurs.

Appliance manufacturers are usually willing to help by giving information about the compounds used in their products so that a suitable appliance that does not incorporate the allergen can be identified.

Dermatological conditions and infections

The peristomal skin is as vulnerable to dermatological conditions such as psoriasis and eczema as the rest of the body. It could be argued that the skin around a stoma is even more susceptible to infections such as candida.

Assessment

1. The nurse should take a detailed history of the condition.
2. The peristomal skin should be examined to determine whether this is a localized or general skin disorder.
3. Swabs should be taken if infection is suspected.

Nursing action

Medical advice must be sought so that the appropriate treatment can be prescribed. Often it is advantageous for the patient to see a dermatologist who may be able to advise on treatments that are non-greasy, thus the adhesion of the appliance will not be compromised. If a greasy application is essential then this must be covered with a waterproof dressing prior to the appliance being applied, for example Opsite^T cut to cover the peristomal skin with an opening just large enough to accommodate the stoma.

In some conditions it may be advisable for the skin to be disturbed as little as possible, and in this case a two-piece appliance may prove advantageous.

COMPLICATIONS SPECIFIC TO ILEAL CONDUIT

Ileal conduits may be prone to the complications previously discussed. However, there are some complications which are specific to this type of urinary stoma.

Infection

To avoid the serious complication of ascending infection into the kidney resulting in pyelonephritis there must be free drainage of urine from the stoma.

If stagnation occurs allowing urine to pool in the conduit then the risk of infection is high. This is often seen when the isolated ileal loop is too long and kinking occurs. Other causes of obstruction are stenosis at skin level or constriction as the conduit passes through the abdominal wall, stricture within the ileal loop or obstruction at the ureteroileal junction due to a calculus or secondary carcinoma. If the urine cannot escape freely it may transmit back pressure to the kidneys.

Intestino-ureteric reflux

Some surgical procedures allow reflux of urine from the conduit back into the ureter to the kidney; this is more common in the ileal conduit than when a loop of colon is used to form the conduit.[10] Some patients naturally have an unusually high intestinal pressure which is capable of forcing urine back into the ureter to the kidney.

Electrolyte reabsorption

The bladder has no absorptive properties but the ileum is 'designed' to absorb. Thus, if a loop of ileum is used to form a conduit for urine, it does not lose this quality and reabsorption of electrolytes destined for excretion can occur. This problem is compounded if the loop of ileum isolated for the conduit is too long, so that urine can linger and stagnate allowing reabsorption to occur.

These three complications may all result in damage to the renal tract which can ultimately result in kidney failure. In serious cases revisional surgery is required to ensure that there is free drainage from the conduit and the urine passes out in minimal time.

Offensive urine

Foul-smelling urine may occur as a result of infection. If this is suspected a sterile specimen should be obtained from the conduit for culture and sensitivity using a fine catheter. If there is proven infection this can then be treated with the appropriate antibiotics.

The patient should be encouraged to take extra fluid. If there is an alteration in the pH of the urine this can also result in odour. A little vinegar in the bag helps to alleviate odour.

Phosphate deposits

Infected or alkaline urine may result in white barnacle-like encrustations forming on a urinary stoma. These deposits cause friction to the stoma resulting in bleeding and providing a portal for further infection to enter, which creates a vicious circle. These deposits may be removed by neutralizing them with an acid substance. Bathing in a solution of 5% acetic acid is often successful. Aci-Jel (Ortho Pharmaceuticals) is a vaginal preparation which contains 0.92% acetic acid in a gel base, and this is also helpful in removing these encrustations. If infection is present Polybactrin spray is a useful preparation to use. High doses (4g daily) of ascorbic acid given daily may also help in treating these encrustations.

Alkaline urine may also result in a blue discolouration of urostomy appliances and night drainage bags. A harmless blue discolouration of the skin may also be noted if a methylcellulose skin protective is used.

CONSTIPATION IN PATIENTS WITH A COLOSTOMY

Normal bowel function is discussed in Chapter 1. Constipation is 'infrequent and undue difficulty in defecation'.[11] What may be considered as normal bowel function in one patient may be grossly abnormal in another. Constipation is only encountered in the patient with a colostomy; failure of an ileostomy to function is usually due to obstruction and is a much more urgent condition.

Possible causes of constipation in the colostomy patient

Dietary

Inadequate or unsuitable diet can result in constipation. Patients who have an inadequate intake of dietary fibre may become constipated; the NACNE (National Advisory Committee on Nutritional Education) report recommended 25–30g daily.[12] The increased intake of over-refined carbohydrate may involve substituting foods high in roughage and cellulose, which will also adversely affect bowel function.

Inadequate fluid intake

Dehydration and inadequate fluid intake can result in larger amounts of water being reabsorbed by the intestine resulting in very dry, hard faeces which are difficult to pass.

Immobility

Hospitalization or incapacitation can restrict the patient's mobility. This, in turn, increases the possibility of constipation as exercise stimulates peristalsis.[13]

Drugs

The most common group of drugs for which constipation is a known side effect is analgesics, particularly opiate derivatives e.g. codeine, morphine and dextropropoxyphene. The constipation results from the effect of these drugs on the smooth muscle of the intestine, reducing peristalsis and prolonging transit time in the bowel.[14] Other drugs that may induce constipation are antacids containing aluminium or calcium as a base, antihypertensive drugs, antidepressants, iron preparations, some diuretics and cytotoxic drugs.

Depression

In depressed and psychotic patients, effects on the hypothalamus and the autonomic nervous system cause inhibition of peristalsis which results in constipation.[15]

Mechanical obstruction

Narrowing of the colonic lumen may be due to recurrence of carcinoma, adhesions or stricture which can cause a slower transit of faeces through the colon.

Age

The elderly are more susceptible to constipation due to increased faecal transit time in the colon[16] and diminished muscle tone[11,15] together with the factors previously mentioned.[13,17,18]

While constipation can affect any patient it can be more difficult to overcome in the patient with a colostomy. If the stoma ceases to function this often causes the patient considerable alarm and his primary worry is often that his disease has recurred or he has a serious disorder.

Treatment of constipation

This primary aim of care is to promote healthy bowel function. The nurse should educate the patient with regard to the importance of eating a diet containing adequate fibre, maintaining an acceptable fluid intake, while encouraging physical mobility.

Laxatives

There are various groups of laxatives which act in different ways and may be indicated for patients with a colostomy who are constipated.

Laxatives that increase bulk. These act by increasing the faecal mass which stimulates peristalsis while also absorbing fluid, thus keeping the faeces moist. These are: bran (Proctofibe or Fybranta, methylcellulose (Celevac or Cellucon), ispaghula husk (Fybogel), sterculia (Normacol). All these are available as proprietary preparations to be taken orally.

Laxatives that increase intestinal motility. These act by decreasing the time the faeces are in the colon thus preventing stasis and hard dry stools. Some examples are: bisacodyl (Dulcolax), danthron (Dorbanex) and senna (Senokot). These preparations can be taken orally and bisacodyl is available as a suppository which has a local stimulant action. These preparations should not be used in intestinal obstruction. Prolonged use should be avoided as they can eventually precipitate the onset of atonic non-functioning colon and hypokalaemia.[19]

Laxatives that attract fluid by osmosis. These are hypertonic and thus attract fluid into the colon; some act more rapidly than others, for instance magnesium sulphate. Others, such as lactulose (Duphalac) is a semisynthetic disaccharide which is not absorbed by the gastrointestinal tract, it produces osmotic diarrhoea. There are also various enema preparations available, such as phosphate enema. One particularly useful preparation is Micralax micro-enema the small volume of which is more easily retained.

Laxatives that soften faeces. These act by softening and lubricating faeces thus facilitating easier defecation, for example docusate sodium (Dioctyl-Medo) which can be taken orally or the liquid preparation may be instilled into the colostomy as a retention enema. Liquid paraffin may be used but can affect the absorption of fat soluble vitamins in prolonged use. There are other oily preparations available for local action, such as arachis oil retention enema.

The patient with a colostomy who develops constipation should be treated in a similar way to any other patient with bowel dysfunction. The local administration of preparations may be less easily achieved due to lack of sphincter muscles to retain the substance. Suppositories often pass back out of the stoma before they have had time to act. Administration of an enema is also problematic as much of the fluid is quickly expelled. Enemas which contain little fluid but are hypertonic are often the most suitable.

If an oil retention enema is required then it may be most easily achieved by inserting a foley catheter well into the stoma and inflating the balloon with up to 5 ml of water; the oil is then instilled via the catheter and the balloon is left inflated for a few minutes after the procedure.[14] If washout of the colostomy is to be performed then the procedure explained in Chapter 15 should be followed using an irrigation cone.

Introduction of any substance into a colostomy must always be preceded by a gentle digital examination to ascertain the direction of the colon. If the substance to be introduced is a liquid it may prove difficult to fit an appliance after the instillation due to the fluid leaking back onto the skin particularly if it is oily. It is often helpful to use a two-piece appliance that clips together for this procedure. (See Chapter 4.) The flange should be affixed to the skin while it is dry and then a drainable bag clipped in place after the enema is given.

If the patient requires regular analgesia as is often the case with those who are terminally ill, then regular prophylactic laxatives should also be prescribed.

The dose of any laxative given to a patient with a colostomy must be carefully monitored and adjusted to prevent the occurrence of diarrhoea which can be equally distressing. Those patients who require regular aperients often prove to be most proficient at regulating their bowel function by adjusting the dose of their medication.

DIARRHOEA

Diarrhoea is the frequent passage of watery motions from the bowel. It should be remembered that the consistency of the faeces passed from the stoma is to a great extent dependent upon the portion of the intestinal tract in which the opening is made. The majority of the fluid is reabsorbed from faeces in the colon. Thus, if a colostomy is created in or distal to the sigmoid colon, the faeces passed should be formed as there has been no compromise of water reabsorption.

Faeces from a colostomy in the transverse colon is usually only semiformed as the reabsorptive function of the colon distal to the stoma has been sacrificed. In the case of an ileostomy the effluent should be of porridge-like consistency but will never be a formed or solid motion because there is no colonic reabsorption of water prior to excretion.

Possible causes of diarrhoea in patients with a stoma

Dietary

Some foods are recognized as being 'natural laxatives' such as fruits, particularly oranges, figs and prunes. In some individuals certain foods will produce diarrhoea that in others will have no effect. Dietary indiscretion is a possible cause of diarrhoea and the patient with a stoma will need to proceed with caution when experimenting with diet. (See Chapter 16.) Some drinks will also induce loose bowel motions such as fruit juices, beer and lager.

Drugs

Antibiotics, particularly those with a relatively broad spectrum of activity such as ampicillin are a well recognized cause of diarrhoea.[20] Other drugs may increase gut motility and result in diarrhoea as a side effect.

Infection

Acute gastroenteritis can be contracted from ingestion of contaminated food or fluids. Infective diarrhoea is usually of mixed aetiology and the onset occurs quite quickly after exposure to the infection.[15] Bacteria such as salmonella, shigella or staphylococcus may be cultured from the stool.

Emotional status

Anxiety may produce heightened reflexes and increased motility, vascularity and rate of mucus secretion in the bowel causing a strong peristaltic rush and frequent evacuation of loose stools.[11] This is due to direct stimulation of the autonomic nervous system.[15]

Disease

The presence of further disease in the intestinal tract can result in diarrhoea. Crohn's disease in particular can cause loose motions but carcinoma or subacute obstruction may also be responsible.

Radiotherapy

If the bowel is included in the treatment area for radiotherapy for example in the case of uterine, ovarian or bladder cancer then severe diarrhoea can result.[21]

Malabsorption

If the gut fails to reabsorb water and digestive products as they pass through the intestine, diarrhoea can result and steatorrhoea may also be noted.

Electrolyte imbalance

If there is a decrease in the body's calcium levels, neuromuscular excitability can occur resulting in hasty elimination.[15]

Treatment of diarrhoea

It is important initially to take a full history and endeavour to ascertain the cause of the diarrhoea. Whatever the cause it is advisable to seek medical advice. Once the cause of the diarrhoea has been elicited, corrective treatment or advice can commence. This may involve dietary advice, counselling, a change in medication or treatment of disease.

Diarrhoea in the patient who has an ileostomy is a potentially serious condition as he can very quickly become dehydrated and suffer electrolyte imbalance, requiring intravenous replacement.

Antidiarrhoeal drugs

Antidiarrhoeal drugs which absorb fluid. Mixtures of chalk and kaolin may be effective in controlling diarrhoea. Methylcellulose and ispaghula husk can also be especially useful in controlling faecal consistency in patients with a colostomy due to their 'mopping up' action on fluids. However, caution should be exercised in patients with an ileostomy, lest dehydration results.

Antidiarrhoeal drugs which reduce motility. Drugs such as codeine phosphate, loperamide (Imodium) and codeine diphenoxylate (Lomotil), all act by reducing the motility of the gut. These drugs are particularly useful for those patients with transverse colostomies and ileostomies. Ideally, the patient should control the dose himself, within certain limits and after instruction, depending upon the nature of his bowel motion. These drugs should not be used in cases of infective diarrhoea as they may delay the passage of liquid faeces, encouraging the proliferation of pathogens and causing the severity of the diarrhoea to be underestimated.[19]

Patients with a colostomy who normally use a closed appliance or manage their stoma by irrigation will need a supply of suitable drainable appliances to avoid the skin becoming damaged by too frequently changing the appliance as a result of more copious bowel effluent. (See Chapter 4.)

Leakage is more likely to occur if the patient develops diarrhoea because watery motion will more readily find a track between the skin and the appliance. A different appliance may need to be selected if the one that the patient normally uses and finds satisfactory is unable to maintain secure adhesion in the presence of large volumes of fluid faeces. Constipation and diarrhoea can affect any patient but in those with a faecal stoma these conditions can be less easy to control and more distressing.

REFERENCES

1. Lister, J., Webster, P.J. & Mirza, S. (1983) Colostomy complications in children. *The Practitioner*, February *227*, 229–237.
2. Devlin, H.B. (1982) Stoma therapy review, part III. *Coloproctology: No. 5.* 298–306.
3. Goligher, J. (1984) *Surgery of the Anus, Rectum and Colon*, 5th edn, Chap. 18, p.568. London: Baillière Tindall.
4. Graham, W.P., Galante, M., Leon, G., McCorkle, H.J. & Wanebo, H.J. (1965) Complications of ileostomy. *American Journal of Surgery, 110*, 142–147.
5. Everett, W.G. (1978) Practical patient care—ileostomies and their problems. *Update, 17*, 205–215.
6. Wilinson, A.J. & Humphries, W.G. (1978) Seat belt injuries to ileostomy. *British Medical Journal, i*, 1249–50.
7. Hinchcliffe, S.M. (1982) The normal function of the alimentary track. In *Stoma Care*. Ed. B. Breckman. Chap. 2, p.40. Beaconsfield: Beaconsfield.
8. Todd, I.P. (1982) Mechanical complications of ileostomy. *Clinics in Gastroenterology, 11*, 268–273.
9. Corman, M.L., Veidenheimer, M.C. & Coller, J.A. (1976) Ileostomy complications: prevention and treatment. In *Contemporary Surgery*, Chap. 8, p.36.
10. Hendry, W.F. (1982) Urinary stomas—surgical procedures and complications. *Clinics in Gastroenterology, 11*, 303–317.
11. Thompson, M. & Bottomley, H. (1980) Normal and abnormal bowel function. *Nursing*, September, *17*, 721–722.
12. National Advisory Committee on Nutritional Education (1983) *NACNE Report*. Health Education Council, London.
13. Pirrie, J. (1980) Constipation in the elderly. *Nursing, 17*, September 753–755.
14. Ainley, R. & Borwell, B. (1984) Constipation—a professional guide. *Nursing Mirror, Supplement, 159*, No. 12.

15. Brooks, S.L. (1984) Disturbances in bowel function. *Nursing, 30*, October 870–876.
16. Brocklehurst, J.C. & Yunis Khan, M. (1969) A study of faecal stasis in old age and the use of Dorbanex in its prevention. *Gerontology Clinics, 11*, 293–300.
17. Anderson, J. (1984) Bowel function in the elderly. *Nursing Times*, 15 August. p.52.
18. Lewin, D. (1976) Care of the constipated patient. *Nursing Times*, 25 March. p.444.
19. *British National Formulary No 8* (1984) London: British Medical Association and The Pharmaceutical Association of Great Britain.
20. Weir, W.R.C. (1984) Diarrhoea, causes and management. *Geriatrics for GPs*. September. 42–46.
21. Breckman, B. (1982) Care of cancer patients with stomas. *Clinics in Gastroenterology, 11*, 397–403.

15   Irrigation technique

The term irrigation describes a procedure for cleansing the bowel by instilling fluid via a stoma. Irrigation via stomas may be carried out for several reasons:

- As a method of management by some colostomy patients to regain faecal continence.
- As a method of cleansing the bowel prior to a procedure, e.g. surgery, X-rays, colonoscopy, etc.
- To empty the bowel of faeces that are causing a problem, e.g. constipation, obstruction.

COLOSTOMY MANAGEMENT BY IRRIGATION

The management of a colostomy by irrigation is not a new technique. It has been practised since the 1920s[1] but there were several reports of patients perforating their colon during the procedure.[2] The other problem was generally poor standards of sanitation, for instance no inside toilet or central heating,[3] thus this method was not recommended. However, with the advent of modern irrigation equipment incorporating a 'cone' for introducing the fluid into the colon the risk of perforation has been reduced.[4] This method of management has now become the one of choice for many patients[5] particularly in the United States.

The aim of colostomy management by irrigation is to restore the patient's continence by enabling him to once more be in control of his bowel function, eliminating faeces only during the irrigation procedure.

Advantages of colostomy management by irrigation

1. The patient regains continence and the need to wear a collecting pouch is therefore avoided; all that is required is a discreet stoma cap or dressing. In many cases this lessens the impact of altered body image and decreases physical and emotional barriers between sex partners.[1]

2. The effects of flatus, diarrhoea and constipation are reduced.[6,7,8]

3. The patient does not have the problem of disposing of soiled appliances.

4. Diet can be more varied and adventuresome with few limitations.[6,8]

5. Patients have reported a better quality of life, improvement in their working lives and sporting and social activities following adoption of this method of colostomy management.[3,6,9]

6. Equipment is available on prescription and will last a considerable time; it is thus an economically viable alternative method of management.[10]

7. The patient does not have to obtain, carry and store regular bulky supplies of appliances and accessories.

8. It is a suitable method of management for patients in hot climates or working in a hot environment where there may be problems with adhesive appliances.

Disadvantages of colostomy management by irrigation

1. The procedure is time consuming and takes approximately one hour.[6] The majority of patients need to irrigate every 48 hours, but some patients need to carry out the procedure daily while a few may manage up to 72 hours between irrigations.[7]

2. The patient may find it difficult to obtain uninterrupted time in the bathroom, particularly if there is only one toilet in the household.

3. The patient may find difficulty in 'improvising' with facilities when away from home.

4. Continual irrigation over a long period of time can result in bowel stasis and natural evacuation may be impaired in the long term.[6]

5. The patient may be unable to continue irrigating in old age and have problems adapting to natural evacuation and wearing an appliance.

6. There is a slight risk of perforating the colon if an inappropriate technique is used.

CHOICE OF PATIENT

The patient who will be suitable to manage his stoma by irrigation must be mentally alert and able to learn the irrigation procedure as well as being physically capable of carrying it out. He must have an 'end' (iliac) colostomy and pass a formed motion. He should also have a normal stoma devoid of any complications, such as stenosis. The patient should also have a good prognosis and there must be no evidence of any further bowel disease, such as diverticular disease.

There must be adequate sanitary facilities at home, ideally a toilet and bathroom combined but a well-heated indoor toilet is a minimum necessity. The patient will also need co-operation from his family since he may have to occupy the bathroom for an hour each day.

The patient himself must have a positive attitude towards the procedure and be well motivated.

Contraindications of colostomy irrigation

1. Patients with right-sided or transverse colostomy where there is a fluid motion, or those in whom the stoma is temporary.
2. Patients with a tendency to diarrhoea which is not controlled by diet or drugs, or those who respond to stress by having diarrhoea.
3. Disease of the remaining colon, such as Crohn's disease as there is a risk of fistula formation, diverticular disease or radiation colitis. Irritable bowel syndrome will also make it inadvisable for the patient to irrigate.
4. There must be caution with patients who have cardiac or renal disease and may have potential fluid overload complications.
5. Stomal complications such as hernia, stenosis or prolapse can make it difficult for the patient to irrigate.
6. Inadequate sanitary facilities or heating at home.
7. Physical or mental limitations of the patient or small children and infants with colostomy.
8. Lack of interest or motivation on the part of the patient in doing the procedure.
9. Nervous or elderly patients to whom the task may prove to be too much of a worry.[8]

PREPARATION OF PATIENT WHO IS TO MANAGE COLOSTOMY BY IRRIGATION

The patient will need careful explanation and counselling about the procedure and what it involves to enable him to make an informed decision. Frank discussion about the advantages and disadvantages of this method of management should take place. It is often helpful to show the patient pictures or slides of somebody irrigating a colostomy so that he can see what is entailed. A video and booklet about irrigation has been recently made for patient education and is an ideal teaching aid.[11] An introduction to a patient with a colostomy who is successfully established on irrigation may also be helpful.

The nurse should check that the procedure would not be contraindicated for any reason and then permission should be sought from the consultant surgeon. The patient's general practitioner should be informed and approval sought. The patient should be shown the irrigation equipment and a range of stoma caps to enable him to choose the type he prefers. A prescription should then be obtained for the equipment and chosen type of cap.

Any modifications to the toilet at home must be discussed. A home visit by the nurse is very helpful to allow her to assess whether the facilities are adequate. Usually all that is required is a hook in the toilet wall which will allow the fluid reservoir to hang with its outlet at shoulder height when the patient is sitting on the toilet (See Fig. 54). When away from home most patients manage to improvise. One method is with a 'lever' suction wall hook which will support the weight of the full fluid reservoir.

The stage at which the patient is taught to irrigate his colostomy is open to debate. Shirley Allen says:

'In America and possibly in some areas of the UK irrigation is taught to patients shortly after surgery. I feel that anybody who has undergone the rigours of an abdominoperineal resection has more than enough to cope with in the early days. This fact, coupled with the lack of adequate conveniences and privacy in hospital, gives every reason for not commencing irrigation for at least 2–3 months following surgery.'[8]

Others also subscribe to this view,[3] as indeed does the author.

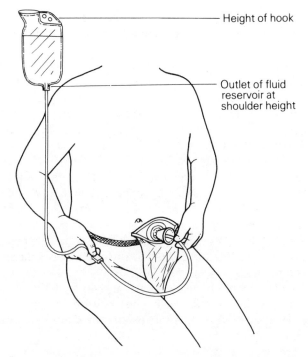

Fig. 54. *Height of hook for suspending fluid reservoir.*

A suitable time for the irrigation should be chosen when the patient can use the facilities of the bathroom undisturbed for about one hour, as a hurried or interrupted irrigation is not conducive to the establishment of intestinal predictability.[12] It does not matter what time is chosen but in one study most patients selected evening.[9]

Teaching the patient to manage his colostomy by irrigation

Ideally, teaching should take place in the patient's own home so that he learns the procedure in the surroundings he is going to be in. The teaching time should preferably be when the patient plans to irrigate regularly. However, if this is not possible some compromise must be discussed.

To allow for adequate teaching the patient will need to be seen daily for at least one week. The procedure should be demonstrated to the patient and each stage clearly explained. The patient should be taught in stages, as with all practical procedures. (See Chapter 10.)

It is essential for the nurse to obtain feedback to ensure that the patient has fully understood her explanations. Written instructions may also prove to be a useful reinforcement. The patient should be advised to continue wearing an appliance between irrigations until continence is established. The period between each irrigation should be extended if there has been no motion via the stoma; the majority of patients find irrigating every 48 hours is adequate. Once the patient has confidence that his colostomy will not act spontaneously he can discard his appliance and wear a discreet stoma cap with flatus filter over his colostomy. (See Chapter 4.) Some patients wear only a piece of lubricated gauze or Melonin. Once the patient is competent he should carry out the procedure unsupervised and the nurse should visit to check his success and advise about any possible problems.

The patient should be made aware of the possibility of colonic perforation, although the nurse must beware of raising undue alarm. The patient should be told clearly the signs and symptoms that can occur and advised to seek medical advice immediately.

THE IRRIGATION PROCEDURE

1. The patient collects and prepares all equipment. (See Fig. 55.) The irrigation cone is attached to the reservoir tubing.
2. The fluid reservoir is filled with one litre of tepid water (approx 37°C).
3. The stoma cap is removed and surrounding skin cleansed.
4. The irrigation bag is placed over the stoma and secured with the belt.
5. The fluid reservoir is hung in a convenient position so that it is within easy reach of the patient and the outlet is level with the patient's shoulder when he sits on the toilet. (See Fig. 54.) *NB* The fluid reservoir must not be too high as this increases the pressure of water entering the bowel. All air is expelled from the tubing by running the water through.
6. The patient sits on the lavatory with the irrigation bag between his legs and passing into the toilet.

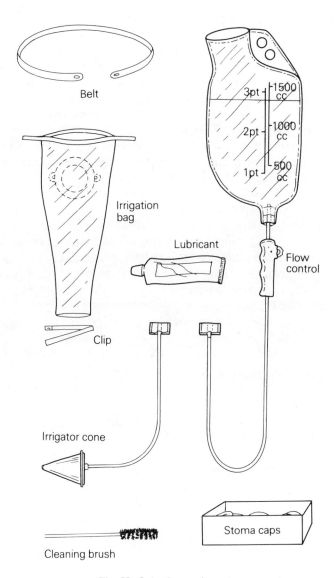

Belt

Irrigation bag

Lubricant

1500 cc
3pt
1000 cc
2pt
500 cc
1pt

Flow control

Clip

Irrigator cone

Stoma caps

Cleaning brush

Fig. 55. *Irrigation equipment.*

7. A gloved finger is introduced into the colostomy to relax the outlet and to assess the direction in which to pass the cone.
8. The cone is lubricated and introduced into the colostomy. *NB The cone must never be removed and the plastic tube pushed into the colon; this increases the risk of perforation.*
9. The fluid is run slowly into the bowel via the colostomy, which should take approximately 20 minutes.
10. Once the reservoir is emptied the cone is removed and the top of the irrigation bag secured.
11. The majority of fluid will be expelled out of the colostomy into the irrigation bag and down the toilet, bring the faecal content in the stream.
12. Once the majority of the fluid is expelled the patient can secure the outlet of the irrigation bag with a clip and move around as desired until the remaining fluid has drained. Privacy is still required as the bag is not discreet, but the time can be utilized for shaving, applying makeup, etc.
13. After about 30 minutes there is no further drainage from the stoma, the irrigation bag is removed, the skin cleansed and dried and a stoma cap or dressing applied.
14. The equipment is then cleansed and stored for future use.

Possible problems and their causes

The fluid will not run into the bowel

1. The cone may not be correctly positioned.
2. The patient may be too tense.
3. The cone may be blocked with faeces.
4. Too much water may be being used.

The water is slow to return

1. The patient may be dehydrated and the water absorbed via the colonic mucosa.
2. Peristalsis may be slow; this may be increased in a variety of ways: moving; coughing sharply; bending from side to side; kneading the abdomen from right to left; drinking hot or cold liquid; pouring lukewarm water over the stoma.

Abdominal cramps

1. The irrigation fluid is running into the bowel too quickly.
2. The irrigation fluid is too hot or too cold.

Bowel acting between irrigations

1. Too long a time between irrigations.
2. Too much water being used which is not expelled.
3. A hurried procedure allowing insufficient time for complete emptying of the bowel.

DISCUSSION

Many patients world-wide now successfully manage their colostomy by regular irrigation as opposed to natural evacuation, although it does not appear to be a popular choice in Great Britian.[13,4] There have been several studies which have indicated the advantages to the patient of this procedure.[3,5,8,9] The ability to predict or control bowel movements for most patients has helped to overcome fears of being 'dirty' and related psychological problems.[7] The equipment is relatively inexpensive (less than the average box of appliances) and can last for a year or more. It is, therefore, a cost-effective method of management particularly for those outside the NHS.

While this method of management is obviously not suited to all patients, and indeed some may find its use distasteful, each patient should be given individual consideration and those who are suitable deserve the opportunity to make their own informed decision.

IRRIGATING A COLOSTOMY AS A METHOD OF PREPARATION FOR A PROCEDURE—PROCEDURE CARRIED OUT BY A NURSE

This procedure should be ordered by a doctor. If the bowel cleansing is prior to surgery antibiotics may be added to the irrigation solution at the surgeon's request. The technique may vary slightly depending upon type of stoma.

End 'iliac' colostomy

Procedure exactly as described as a method of colostomy management.

Loop colostomy

There are two types of irrigation.

Distal washout

Fluid is run into the distal opening in the colostomy using an irrigation set and cone. The fluid then passes along the colon distal to the colostomy and is passed by the patient per rectum. (See Fig. 56.) The procedure is carried out as previously described. However, little irrigation fluid will be expelled into the irrigation bag as the majority will pass directly into the lavatory.

It is important to identify the distal opening in the colostomy. Anatomically this should be to the left of the stoma but it may be twisted so digital examination of both openings should reveal faeces in the proximal colon and mucus only in the distal loop. Alternatively the patient may well be able to identify the active

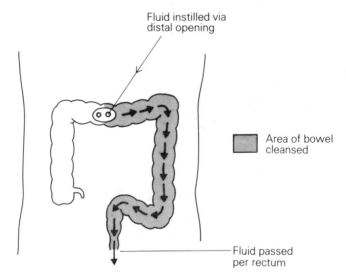

Fluid instilled via distal opening

Area of bowel cleansed

Fluid passed per rectum

Fig. 56. *Area cleansed by distal washout of a loop colostomy.*

outlet. This procedure is contraindicated in cases where the patient has an obstructing lesion. Fluid should only be run into the colon very slowly until patency is established. When fluid is passed per rectum the rate can then be increased.

Proximal washout

Fluid is run into the proximal opening in the colostomy using an irrigation set and cone. The fluid passed into the colon proximal to the colostomy is then expelled via the colostomy together with any bowel motion in the colon. (See Fig. 57.)

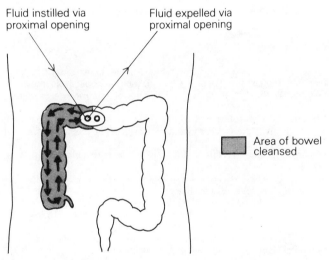

Fluid instilled via proximal opening

Fluid expelled via proximal opening

Area of bowel cleansed

Fig. 57. *Area cleansed by proximal washout of a loop colostomy.*

The procedure is carried out as described in the method to manage a colostomy by irrigation. Care must be taken not to run too much fluid at once into the proximal colon or to introduce the fluid under pressure as this may cause backwash past the ileocaecal valve into the sterile ileum.

Loop ileostomy

Irrigation of an ileostomy should only be performed by an experienced nurse. The procedure is as for a loop colostomy except that a *fine soft rubber catheter* may be used instead of a cone.

IN CASES OF OBSTRUCTION

If the ileostomy is obstructed, a washout is usually only attempted following abdominal X-rays and a medical opinion. Small amounts (approximately 30 ml) of sterile normal saline solution are introduced into the ileostomy and no further fluid is instilled until this is returned.

If a colostomy has not functioned due to the patient being constipated, warm oil or dioctyl sodium succinate solution in warm water may be instilled to soften the faeces prior to irrigation.

REFERENCES

1. Aylett, S. (1978) Colostomy care by washout (or irrigation) technique. In *Intestinal Stomas*. Ed. Todd, I. Chap. 6, p.60. London: Heinemann.
2. Gabriel, W.B. (1927) Discussion on colostomy. *Proceedings of the Royal Society of Medicine, 20*, 1452.
3. Williams, N.S. & Johnson, D. (1980) Prospective controlled trial comparing colostomy irrigation with spontaneous evacuation method. *British Medical Journal*, 12 July. 107.
4. Griffiths, & Shorey, (1978) Modern colostomy management. *Update*, 1 January. 105–114.
5. Stockley, A. (1981) Irrigation. In *Stoma Care*. Ed. Breckman, B., Chap. 11. p.140. Beaconsfield: Beaconsfield.
6. Colostomy Welfare Group (1982) *Irrigation, 13*, April.
7. Terranova, A. et al. (1979) Irrigation v. natural evacuation of left colostomy. *Diseases of Colon and Rectum*. January/February, 31–4.
8. Allan, S. (1984) Stoma management. *Nursing, 30*, 877–881.
9. Phillpotts, E.A., Griffiths, D.A., Eltringham, W.K. & Espiner, H.J. (1976) The continent colostomy. *Nursing Mirror*, 20 May. 53–4.
10. Devlin, H.B. (1982) Stoma therapy—review II. *Coloproctology*, pp.8–17.
11. Evans, B.D., French, C.M.A. & Fahey, K. (1984) *'So You've Heard About Irrigation...'*. Available from Royal College of Nursing, London.
12. Mazier, Dignam, Capehart, & Smith, (1976) The surgeon at work 'effective colostomy irrigation'. *Surgery, Gynaecology and Obstetrics*, June *142*, 905–9.
13. McDonald, L., Anderson, H.R., & Bennett, A.E. (1982) *Cancer Patients in the Community: Outcomes of Care and Quality of Survival in Rectal Cancer*. Report submitted to DHSS (June 1982) HMSO, London.

16 Other considerations in stoma care

DIET

All patients who have a stoma will require advice about their diet, and when discussing the dietary implications there are two basic considerations to be made:

- The dietary needs of the individual to avoid any nutritional deficiency.
- The possible effects of certain foods on stomal function.

Patients with a stoma require a well-balanced, varied diet to provide them with the nutrients they need. It has been suggested that nearly half the patients in Britain who have major abdominal surgery suffer from malnutrition.[1] It is therefore essential that the nutritional status of the patient is monitored before and after surgery and any deficiences are corrected.

Ileostomy patients may be liable to develop water and salt depletion due to the greater volume of effluent passed and the limited ability of the ileum to conserve sodium. In most cases ileostomy patients do not have any clinical symptoms but chronic dehydration may be indicated by blood tests.[2] If further losses of water and salt occur due to a condition such as gastroenteritis, severe depletion can quickly occur. This may also be the case if the patient sweats excessively and those in hot climates may need fluid and salt replacement.

There are three situations in which ileostomy patients are particularly prone to dehydration due to excessive loss:

1. Immediately postoperatively when the ileostomy may produce large volumes of effluent.
2. Ileostomy dysfunction which results in high volumes of effluent.
3. Removal of the terminal ileum which is the major site where sodium conservation occurs.

Ileostomy patients may experience cramps due to salt depletion which respond to replacement therapy. In some cases the cramps may be due to a deficiency of magnesium or calcium thus these trace elements should also be replaced. 'Although all ileostomy patients are at risk from water and salt depletion when losses are increased above normal, very few require regular replacement.'[3]

In cases where part of the small intestine has been excised malabsorption may occur. This may result in the patient requiring digestive supplements and adjusting their dietary intake of certain foodstuffs, such as fats. If it is not possible for the patient to maintain his nutritional status due to extensive intestinal resection he may require nutritional support administered either enterally or parenterally. However, it is suggested that the remaining small bowel undergoes adaptive changes to increase its absorptive capacity for a period of up to two years.[3]

Research suggests that the majority of patients with a stoma have no difficulty in selecting a suitable diet.[4,5] The majority tend to avoid one or two items of food only, while a few exclude certain foods from their diet completely.[4] The foods which patients with a stoma tend to avoid are those which may result in socially embarrassing consequences, such as flatus, fluid effluent or odour, although many patients find odour is less of a problem now that appliances are made from odourproof materials.[4]

The foods which patients with a colostomy have identified as the most troublesome are:

- Odour—Green vegetables, onions.
- Flatus—Green vegetables, onions, fruit.
- Fluid effluent—Fruit, green vegetables.

While those with an ileostomy have reported the following:[4]

- Odour—Fish, eggs, onions.
- Flatus—Peas, onions, beans, fizzy drinks.
- Fluid effluent—Fruit, vegetables, fish.[4,5]

It is possible that green vegetables produce a smell in patients with a colostomy due to the action of colonic bacteria. However, some patients with ileostomies also complain of odour after eating greens and this may be due to bacterial colonization of the terminal ileum.[3]

Some patients with a stoma find that alcoholic drinks, particularly beer, result in a fluid effluent. It is not possible to give patients with a stoma rigid dietary instruction since the foods that cause problems for one individual may prove totally acceptable to another. The patient should be advised to introduce new foods into his diet gradually so that he can identify the 'culprit' if stoma dysfunction occurs. However, if he does decide to eat a particular food that he knows causes problems on occasion, deeming the dysfunction to be an acceptable price to pay for enjoyment, then he is well advised to eat these foods when he knows that he will have the facilities available to cope with any problems. It is obviously not ideal to eat foods which produce excessive fluid effluent prior to taking a long bus journey! It may also be necessary to use a different appliance, such as a drainable bag, or incorporate a flatus filter if dysfunction occurs. Most ileostomy patients find that the greatest volume of effluent is passed three to four hours after their main meal, hence this is usually in the evening. Patients with a colostomy, however, usually find that their first meal of the day stimulates bowel action, thus the colostomy usually functions in the morning. These timings may need to be considered by the patient when selecting his diet.

Patients who have an ileostomy should be cautioned regarding the risk of obstruction if large quantities of high residue foods are eaten and not adequately chewed. It is therefore essential that an ileostomist who does not have a full set of teeth has correctly fitting dentures to enable him to chew his food. Some foods may be described as indigestable by ileostomists and are recognizable after excretion, for example nuts. Beetroot may cause red discoloration of ileostomy effluent. These occurrences may be alarming to new patients.[6] Eating out is a popular social pastime for many patients and one that they should be encouraged to resume. Some patients may initially be reluctant to go out and eat. This is usually due to anxiety about selecting from a restaurant menu or fears of stoma dysfunction during the meal. It may be helpful if the patient approaches these difficulties in stages until he has regained his confidence. For example, it is often better to go out initially with a very close relative or friend who knows about the stoma. It may also be helpful to go to a restaurant which offers a wide variety of foods so that selection from the menu is less difficult. Visiting the home of an acquaintance whose wife has obviously spent hours preparing an exotic meal may be disastrous if the patient is unsure of what to eat but finds refusing the food embarrassing.

It is wise to inform patients of foods that may result in stoma dysfunction so that they can exercise a degree of caution. Also, dietary advice must reflect economic reality as it is often the more expensive foods that create least dysfunction. However, all stoma patients should be encouraged to eat as varied a diet as possible and should try foods that cause dysfunction two or three times before deciding to exclude them from their diet.[3,4,5]

Cultural and religious implications on diet

Patients from different cultures observe varying dietary restrictions, some of which are shown in the following chart.

Religion	Foods avoided	Other considerations
Muslim	Pork, lard or animal fat from pigs. Alcohol. May avoid European hard cheese due to the strong flavour. Any meat or meat product which is not halal.	Beef, mutton, chicken and fats from these animals are eaten provided the animal has been slaughtered in a specific way (halal meat) i.e. allowed to bleed to death and dedicated to Allah by a Muslim.
Sikh	Beef, lard or animal fat from cattle. May avoid European hard cheese due to the strong flavour. Some Sikhs avoid pork, considering it to be unclean.	Some Sikhs are strict vegetarians, thus all meat and animal fats are avoided.
Hindu	Beef and pork or animal fats from pigs or cattle.	Some Hindus avoid mutton, chicken, fish and all animal fat. Very strict Hindus do not eat eggs.
Jewish	Pork, lard or animal fats from pigs. Any meat or meat product that is not kosher.	All meat eaten by Jews must be killed in a certain way (kosher) so that the blood drains away. Jews are forbidden to eat meat and dairy products together as part of the same meal.

The nurse must consider these restrictions when offering the patient dietary advice. She should also ascertain the main sources of protein in the diet since in some cases to restrict vegetable intake in a bid to reduce flatus could result in malnutrition.

Many Asian and Oriental patients dislike hospital food intensely, finding it tasteless, heavy and unpleasant in texture.[7]

Patients often refuse food in case it contains forbidden ingredients. Food that has been in contact with forbidden food is also unacceptable as it is contaminated. A patient cannot eat salad from which a slice of meat has been removed because all the food on the plate is then considered contaminated; similarly vegetables served with meat gravy are unacceptable. Many patients from ethnic groups will need help in selecting from a menu as they are frequently unfamiliar with Western titles such as 'shepherd's pie' or 'Irish stew' and will not know what ingredients these foods contain.

Some foods may be considered by the patient to be beneficial to health, for instance the Chinese often consider rice is the only form of food that can give them energy or vitality. A traditional Chinese belief is that soup boiled for six to seven hours will help clear the system and promote speedy recovery, particularly after surgical operations.[8]

Often the patient's family will be willing to bring food into the hospital for him. In this case they should be informed of any dietary restrictions made on medical grounds. This may be advantageous in encouraging the patient to eat, as a strange diet is even less appetizing if one is ill; it is familiar food that is most likely to be eaten.

Some religious groups such as Muslims, Jews and Buddhists fast on certain occasions, which may involve abstaining from eating any food for several hours or eating only certain foods such as fruit or yoghurt or nuts. Medication may also be refused when fasting. These practices can result in severe stomal dysfunction and this must be explained to the patient, particularly if he has an ileostomy. Some foods eaten on religious occasions may also cause problems with bowel function, such as 'Mazza', the traditional unleavened Passover bread eaten by Jews during the seven-day Passover holiday. This can lead to diarrhoea in some cases, constipation in others.[9] In most religions patients may be exempted from fasting on health grounds. However, some devout patients who break food restrictions may feel sinful, disgusted and very distressed.[7]

Some families have been reported to be reluctant to accept food prepared by a person with a stoma, due to the relationship of the stoma on the abdomen facing the food being prepared.[10]

IMPLICATIONS OF CULTURAL AND RELIGIOUS BELIEFS ON STOMA CARE

The nursing process advocates individualized nursing care and when making a nursing assessment the patient's cultural and religious beliefs must be considered.

'All patients should be treated as individuals and their health care related to their way of life. It is important for the nurse to understand something of the culture and way of life of those patients who belong to ethnic minorities if their health care is to be successful. All ethnic groups have different cultures and these differences should be understood by all those involved in health care.'[11]

When discussing stoma care it is essential to consider the patient as a whole. The information in this section is intended to give a general understanding of the difficulties faced by patients from ethnic minority groups. The fact that these patients have a stoma can cause many additional cultural difficulties.

The three major ethnic groups present in the United Kingdom are Asian, West Indian and Chinese.[10] In the 1981 census 4.1% of the total population consisted of racial minorities, of whom 57% were of Asian origin. For the nurse, 'To enter the cultural and religious world of a patient whose background is different from one's own can be bewildering and difficult.'[10]

Ethnic minorities in the United Kingdom generally live in working class, inner city areas.[11] Their housing conditions are often overcrowded which results in a lack of privacy. This can make caring for a stoma particularly difficult.

Differences in language can often hamper communication between staff and patient. Whenever possible a member of staff who has a good command of English and the patient's language should be asked to interpret. If this is not possible then the local minority community, the community relations council or other local organizations for minority groups may be able to provide an interpreter.[8] Nurses must be sensitive to communication barriers and clearly explain procedures in simple language. The use of pictorial language cards may also be helpful. The nurse should also be aware and respond to non-verbal communication and signals of distress and confusion. However, even with an efficient interpreter counselling can prove very difficult.

The incidence of disease which predisposes to surgery involving the formation of a stoma is often quite low within ethnic minority groups, possibly due to their diet. Thus those who do have a stoma are likely to become isolated within their culture. In their country of origin the number of hospital beds available is low compared to the population and they are used only for the seriously ill;[1] therefore, the patient may be extremely anxious on admission to hospital and fear he is dying; this can compound language and cultural difficulties.

Some patients from minority groups may prefer to return to their own country for treatment which may appear strange to Western health care workers. However, if one imagines oneself taken ill in a Third World country then one's own reactions may be similar! Some patients may delay seeking treatment relying initially on home remedies and herbal medicine. This can often result in disease being very advanced when the patient presents for treatment.

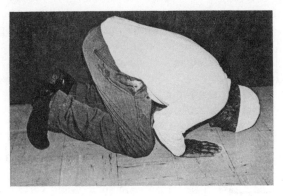

Fig. 58 *A Muslim praying.*

Religious and cultural beliefs should also be considered when siting the stoma preoperatively. Some groups wear trousers or saris which concentrate bulk at waist level. Muslims' prayer rituals require them to prostrate themselves (Sujud). (See Fig. 58.) Faeces are often considered unclean thus some patients may find a stoma placed above the waistline more acceptable, associating the effluent more with ingested food than faecal elimination.

Cultural beliefs

The creation of a stoma may be viewed by some patients as a punishment and/or seen as evidence of a wrong-doing in a previous life.[10] In addition, the rituals of culture or religion may make it difficult for a patient to adapt to life with a stoma.

An important part of Jewish life is the Sabbath which lasts from sunset on Friday to sunset on Saturday. Some Jews observe their day of rest strictly and are reluctant to perform any tasks, even caring for their stoma. Jewish religious law releases the sick from these stringent rules but the pious may find management of a colostomy by irrigation on alternate days more acceptable.[9] However, any danger of life overrules all religious laws.

The Muslim prays five times each day and is required to carry out a ritual cleansing under running water. The patient will also require a clean stoma appliance at this time and for this a two-piece system is often more suitable as it avoids skin damage resulting from frequent changing. The appliance must also be secure to avoid leakage during prostration (kneeling and touching the forehead to the ground) and the use of a belt may be helpful. Prayers take place on clean ground facing Mecca; if the patient is too ill and physically unable to adopt this position he may pray silently in bed provided he is clean and the bed faces Mecca (south east in Britain).

Arab and Pakistani men will often be reluctant to accept instructions from a female nurse or doctor.[9] This is because in their culture women are inferior and this may cause a difficulty for the nurse trying to teach self-care of the stoma. Some religions observe a 'caste-system' believing individuals are born into the caste for which his behaviour in a past life has fitted him. Members of each caste have a certain role in society and certain duties to perform.[12] Some Asians hold rigid views and caste differences have an important effect on acceptance thus it is vital when selecting a visitor with a stoma for a patient that their caste and that of the visitor is considered. It should be remembered also that Sikhs regard bodily hair as sacred and the hair should not be cut or shaved unless this is unavoidable.[7]

Family

Many patients from ethnic minorities come from an extended family, thus they are cared for by the family who will also take over their responsibilities such as care of children while they are ill. Asian cultures are patriarchal but West Indian society is matriarchal, with men playing a less dominant role.[10] The oldest member of the household is usually considered as head of the family and, when any major decisions are discussed, the final decision is made by the older members of the family—men in particular.[1] This is usually the case when the decision to undergo surgery is taken. It may therefore be necessary to include the family head in preoperative explanations. Some patients may also discuss this decision with their religious leader.

Some male patients may expect their wives to care for their stoma and in some families this is acceptable. Asians have very close family ties and they find it difficult to understand if they cannot stay with the patient most of the time to console and care for him, as happens in Asian hospitals.[13] It can be distressing to the patient and his family if they must adhere to restricted visiting hours. The patient with a stoma who cannot understand Western hospital rules may conclude he is being ostracized from his family.

Cleanliness

Many cultures reserve the right hand for 'clean' tasks only, such as eating and greeting. The left hand is used to wash the pubic and anal area. The patient may wish to change his stoma appliance using only his left hand and a suitable appliance should be sought. A two-piece clip-on bag may prove to be the most suitable. Alternatively, the patient may use disposable plastic or rubber gloves.

Most Asian patients prefer to wash in running water and will refuse a bath, considering sitting in dirty water unacceptable. This may be a problem if the patient has a perineal wound to cleanse in which case use of a shower with a movable nozzle or a bidet may be the solution.

Modesty

Patients from ethnic minority groups are in many cases very modest and will have great difficulty accepting being in a mixed ward. They may be extremely reluctant to undress even in front of a member of the same sex. Most Asian women much prefer to be cared for and examined by a female nurse or doctor. Men may also be very uncomfortable if they are undressed in the presence of a female.

Bowel function may be considered to be private and the patient may learn self-care very quickly, finding it unbearable for the nurse to deal with such a private function. Conversely, some patients may be reluctant to learn, viewing bag changing as a medical matter.[10]

Attitude to illness

The emotional reaction to illness varies, some cultures expecting the patient to face his illness with stoicism and emotional control while others expect the patient to react emotionally to his illness.[14] As stomas are a rarity amongst patients of Asian origin this may influence their attitudes. When Asians are ill they are expected to fit the sick role in their society and concepts such as early ambulation and rehabilitation may not be understood.[10]

'The concept of a professional who "cares" in a personal way is alien and contradictory to most people brought up in an Asian culture.'[12] The family may find it threatening if the nurse visits the patient at home unless the purpose of such visits have been clearly explained. When visiting the home the nurse should show respect to the elders of the family and greet them as they will judge her attitude towards them by her behaviour. In some cases it may be difficult to gain entry to the home as a husband may instruct his wife not to open the door in his absence or a woman who speaks little English may find it easier to pretend she is not in than to feel humiliated by her inability to converse.[12]

Other potential problems are that the family may mistrust the nurse if they consider her clothing immodest by their standards, and if women are considered inferior a wife may not speak while her husband or elders are present.

Hospitality plays an important part in some cultures and when visiting the nurse may be offered food and drink, which it is good manners to accept.[12]

Sex and marriage

Some cultures still arrange marriages for their children. The presence of a stoma will be considered as a serious imperfection which will result in a less satisfactory match being made. Loss of fertility or potency will also be regarded as a major disaster as traditional Asian culture places overwhelming importance on children, especially sons. If a woman cannot have children she may feel she has failed as a wife.

Discussion of sexual activity or problems is often not acceptable to Asian patients who view this aspect of their lives as very personal.

Sexual intercourse is a 'Mitzvah' (command) that a Jewish husband pledges in the contract of marriage to fulfil with certain minimal frequency. If the male Jew becomes impotent after stoma surgery he will often seek a penile implant to help him overcome his psychosocial inhibitions and perform his religious sexual duties.[9]

Some nurses who are from different cultures may experience difficulties in caring for patients who have a stoma. If this is the case the nurse should seek advice and counselling from her tutor or a nurse counsellor. It is important that the nurse is aware that her own cultural values will influence the advice she gives.

It is essential that the nurse is able to empathize with the patient with a stoma if the care she gives is to be satisfactory. The nurse must respect the religious practices of the patient if their caring relationship is not to be damaged. 'A cultural gap may remain unbridged for ever with resultant lifelong suffering for the ostomist unless the carer can enter his world.'[10]

This information is intended to guide nurses who are caring for patients with a stoma who are from different cultures and religions. More specific information is beyond the scope of this book. Further help is often available from a hospital chaplain or minister and further reading is suggested below.

Further reading

1. Henley, A. (1979) *Asian Patients in Hospital and At Home.* King Edward's Hospital Fund. Pitman Medical Press.
2. *Religions and Cultures—A guide to Patient's Beliefs and Customs for Health Service Staff.* (1978) Compiled by Lothian Community Relations Council, Scotland.
3. Henley, A. (1983) *Caring for Sikhs and Their Families: Religious Aspects of Care.* Produced for the DHSS and the King Edward's Hospital Fund for London by the National Extension College.
4. Henley, A. (1983) *Caring for Hindus and Their Families: Religious Aspects of Care.* Produced for the DHSS and the King Edward's Hospital Fund for London by the National Extension College.
5. Henley, A. (1983) *Caring for Moslems and Their Families: Religious Aspects of Care.* Produced for the DHSS and the King Edward's Hospital Fund for London by the National Extension College.
6. McDermott, M.Y. & Ahsan, M.M. (1980) *The Muslim Guide.* The Islamic Foundation.

SEXUAL IMPLICATIONS OF STOMA SURGERY

Many patients who have undergone surgery which leaves them with an abdominal stoma experience sexual difficulties after their operation.[15,16] These problems may be the result of physiological or psychological disturbances.[17] 'In social and sexual situations the ostomate feels vulnerable. Will it leak? Will it smell? Will it make noises? Will their partner be disgusted?'[18] Physiological sexual problems result in patients following rectal excision if damage to the nerves supplying the sexual organs occurs or if pelvic anatomy is altered.

Some patients who have an ileostomy created after a long period of illness may find that as their general health improves so does their libido. Some females report that their sexual activity before operation was curtailed due to general malaise, diarrhoea, abdominal pain and fear of incontinence.[19] A survey of ileostomy patients revealed that while 36% of patients reported a change in pattern of intercourse this was a negative change for only 28%, representing a positive change for some couples.[15]

It appears that marital breakdown amongst couples where one partner has a stoma is no more prevalent than in the rest of the population. However, if a marriage is already shaky then the stoma may be a good excuse for ending it altogether.[20] Research amongst a group of 409 patients with a stoma indicated that surgery did not alter the habits of masturbation, petting and premarital sex but showed a decline in extramarital sexual activity.[21]

Physiological problems

It is suggested that impotence occurs in 28%–29% of male patients following rectal excision for cancer;[22] the incidence appears to increase with the patient's age at operation. When surgery to remove the rectum is performed for ulcerative colitis the incidence of impotence is less, being 25% at the most.[22]

Pelvic nerve damage is less common when the rectum is removed for ulcerative colitis since only the rectal wall and rectal mucosa need to be removed and thus adjacent structures can be preserved in the majority of cases. When the rectum is excised to remove a malignancy then a greater amount of tissue is removed, this may cause the sympathetic and parasympathetic nerve supply to the bladder and sexual organs to be sacrificed in an attempt to remove the cancer.[17]

In the male patient damage to the sympathetic presacral nerve will result in the inability to ejaculate although he will still be able to achieve an erection. If the parasympathetic nerves (nervi errigentes) are damaged then the patient will experience erectile difficulties. It is recognized that male patients who experience difficulty in emptying their bladder postoperatively often experience sexual problems later.[23]

In female patients excision of the rectum often results in an alteration of pelvic anatomy, a change in the angle of the vagina and perineal scarring. Pelvic sepsis may predispose to the development of adhesions across the vagina. In some women a lack of vaginal elasticity may prevent their partner's penis being gripped adequately during intercourse. Women may also notice a deficiency in lubrication which can make intercourse uncomfortable. Discharge of mucus from a retained rectum may also cause embarrassment to some female patients during intercourse.

Some male patients who have a colostomy have reported that defecation occurs when they achieve orgasm, and this is thought to be due to increased autonomic nervous activity.[23]

Chemotherapy, radiation and analgesics are all associated with generalized feelings of malaise. This can have a profound effect on feelings of self-esteem, sexuality and libido.[24] These factors should be taken into consideration as they can compound the sexual difficulties experienced by patients who have a stoma.

Psychological problems

The creation of an abdominal stoma represents an alteration in body image which can result in the patient having a poor self-concept and reduced self-esteem. The patients often perceive themselves to be less attractive sexually to their partner. Research suggests that this is the case in about 50% of patients with ileostomies, while only 9% of husbands and 6% of wives are reported to agree with this view.[25]

Poor self-concept and lack of self-esteem may lead the patient to fear his partner's infidelity or rejection. This can create a vicious circle in which the patient, seeing himself as being less sexually desirable, avoids intimate contact with his partner. The partner, being unsure of how to express her continued love, and hesitant to make an advance lest it damage the stoma or cause pain, accepts the situation without comment. This then serves to reinforce the patient's perceptions of being undesirable.

Patients who have an established relationship will often benefit from having their partner to support them through their surgery. However, it should be remembered that the patient who fears rejection has, in fact, got 'something to lose'—a loved one whom they have grown close to. Single patients face the problem of telling a prospective partner about their stoma. This is usually best accomplished early in a relationship before an emotional investment has been made; rejection at this stage is often less traumatic. Patients should be advised that honesty is the best policy and that disclosure is preferable to discovery. Acceptance of the stoma by the partner is often gradual and frank discussion is important.

Impotence may occur as a result of psychological rather than physiological factors. Performance-anxiety and fear of failure often lead to actual failure and the problem becomes self-perpetuating. It may be distressing for a man to accept that his difficulty has a psychological basis.[26] Psychological influences may also predispose to physiological problems in a woman. If a woman fears intercourse will be painful she is often anxious, hence little genital lubrication is produced and penetration by the penis is difficult. This results in dyspareunia.

The patient may be in need of information and reassurance about sexual activity after surgery. Ideally, the subject should be discussed before they leave hospital. The patient should be told that while fear of failure is common and understandable, severe anxiety may prevent satisfactory sexual relationships, and it is therefore important to maintain a sense of balance. Reassurance should be given that sexual activity will not damage the stoma provided it is not used as an orifice, nor should sex be painful once recovery from surgery has occurred. It is inadvisable for the patient to rush into resuming sexual activity; he should wait until he feels comfortable. Some patients prefer to avoid foods which they can identify as causes of stoma dysfunction for several hours prior to sex, although this may not be practical as sexual encounters often occur spontaneously.

The nurse may also be able to make some practical suggestions which the patient may find helpful. It is advisable that the appliance is emptied immediately prior to sex so that pressure does not result in leakage. Opaque bags may be more acceptable to the patient and their partner. Many patients prefer to wear an appliance cover which disguises the pouch. The bag may be rolled up into a smaller shape and taped down so that it does not flap and its presence becomes negligible.[27] It may be more acceptable to some patients to wear a smaller bag for intimate times and some colostomists who have a regular bowel habit may wear only a stoma cap. (See Chapter 4.) Some female patients make very attractive feminine covers to match their underwear. (See Fig. 59.) Other patients prefer to disguise the appliance by wearing attractive open crotch panties.

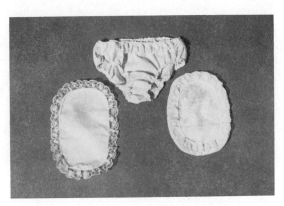

Fig. 59. *Attractive appliance covers.*

Female patients who experience dyspareunia or fear that deep penetration may cause them pain often find a change of sexual position advantageous. If the angle of the vagina is altered, intercourse with both partners lying on their sides may be more comfortable. Women who experience deep dyspareunia in the traditional 'missionary' position may feel more in control if intercourse takes place with her in the superior position, on top of her partner. If lack of natural lubrication is a problem a substitute lubricant such as KY jelly or saliva may be an acceptable alternative.

A satisfying sexual relationship does not necessarily have to include intercourse. The patient may benefit from suggestions of methods of alternative gratification, such as mutual masturbation or oral sex. Some individuals may need reassuring that no sexual practice which provides pleasure and satisfaction to those concerned without harm to themselves or others can justifiably be regarded as wrong or evil.[25]

Sexual aids

Some patients regard manufactured aids with suspicion or feel that their use would be unacceptable, while others accept them quite readily. Thus tactful discretion must be used if their use is to be suggested.

There are a variety of products available which may be helpful to patients experiencing physiological sexual difficulties such as: penile implants; energizing rings which pulsate and improve an erection; and devices which impede penile return to help maintain an erection. Female patients with diminished sensitivity may get greater satisfaction if their partner wears a ring over his penis with small protrusions which stimulate the labia and clitoris. Artificial penises or vaginas which strap to the body are also available. A vibrator may be effective in enhancing sensation and facilitating orgasm.

Many of these products are available by mail order as well as being on sale in sex shops. Advice about purchase is available from Association for Sexual and Personal Relationships of the Disabled. (See Chapter 12.)

Pregnancy

In some female patients who have had severe pelvic sepsis associated with their disease, fertility may be impaired due to obstruction of the fallopian tubes. In such cases in vitro fertilization may be considered.

Many patients who have a stoma have had successful pregnancies. However, as the abdomen distends and stretches the stoma may be hidden from view, and the patient may then need a mirror to enable her to change her appliance. The patient sometimes requires a different appliance as leakage may occur due to changes in the abdominal contours, fetal movement, or retraction of the stoma if it is under tension as the uterus enlarges.

Intestinal obstruction may occur in pregnant patients if changes in the peritoneum result in adhesions becoming taut around the intestine.

Vaginal delivery is usually possible for patients who have had ulcerative colitis.[29] However, forceps delivery may be required.[30] An extended episiotomy is often needed to prevent tearing of the previously scarred perineum. In patients who have had Crohn's disease delivery is often achieved by Caesarian section as an episiotomy may not heal well and fistula formation can occur.

Contraception

Contraceptive advice is often required by female patients who have a stoma. It is possible that the contraceptive pill will not be fully absorbed, particularly if the patient has intestinal hurry or some of the small bowel has been resected. The low dose pill is, therefore, particularly unsuitable.

As previously discussed surgery can result in altered pelvic anatomy, which may make the use of a Dutch cap very difficult for the patient. Intrauterine contraceptive devices (IUD) can also be difficult to insert and an anaesthetic may be required. If pelvic infection is a problem this method of contraception is contraindicated.[31]

Sterilization at the time of surgery may be considered for a woman whose family is complete. However, when the woman is unwell and contemplating life with a stoma, her ability to make such a permanent decision is impaired. Sterilization at a later date is not advised, particularly via a laproscope since adhesions will make the procedure difficult and there is an increased risk of damaging the intestine.[31]

Depo-Provera which is administered by injections at three-monthy intervals may be a suitable method of contraception for some female patients, otherwise she may have to rely on her partner to take contraceptive precautions.

Some male patients who have undergone rectal excision find using a sheath unacceptable as it reduces sensation, which may already be impaired due to nerve damage during surgery.

Homosexuality

Rectal excision is particularly distressing to a homosexual as it may result in curtailment of his sexual activity and his being forsaken by his 'gay' friends. The patient must be warned that the stoma must not be used as an orifice for intercourse as this will result in damage to the bowel. Venereal disease and AIDS can be transmitted via a stoma in this way.[30] If it is not acceptable to the partner to enjoy alternative means of gratification other than anal intercourse he should seek another consort. Such an arrangement is often acceptable within a 'gay' community with the stoma patient not feeling jealous provided the emotional relationship remains intact.[28]

It is essential that patients who have a stoma are given the help and support they require to enable them to resume a satisfying sexual relationship. Sensitive counselling is of paramount importance and aspects of sexual counselling are discussed in Chapter 6. The patient's partner should be involved in his care throughout, so that the couple can accept any changes together. It may be helpful if patients can ask the stoma care nurse or doctor to talk to a new partner and offer explanations if this situation arises. Patients who have complex sexual difficulties which are beyond the scope of the nurse's skills should be sensitively referred to the appropriate expert.

There are various leaflets available which offer valuable information to patients with stomas and can reinforce professional advice. Some patients may find open discussion of such a personal aspect of their lives extremely difficult in which case reading may be a more acceptable way of getting information.

Useful leaflets

1. *Sex Courtship and the Single Ostomate.* United Ostomy Association Inc.
2. *Sex and the Female Ostomate.* United Ostomy Association Inc.
3. *Sex Pregnancy and the Female Ostomate.* United Ostomy Association Inc.
4. *Sex and the Male Ostomate.* United Ostomy Association Inc.
5. *Sex and the Person with an Ostomy.* Association for the Sexual and Personal Relationships of the Disabled. (See Chapter 12.)

TRAVEL AND HOLIDAYS

Travelling or going away for a holiday may present some anxiety to a patient who has a stoma. If the patient is planning a trip away and is in any way unsure he should seek advice from his stoma care nurse, doctor or stoma association. The important thing is for patients with a stoma to feel confident in travelling a distance and to feel sure they have suitable accommodation to use when they arrive at their destination.

Coping with the appliance away from home

It is advisable for patients to carry a small emergency kit with them at all times. This should contain a spare appliance (prepared for use) and a means of cleansing the skin. Small sachets of impregnated tissue (Stoma-wipes) are available for purchase and are ideal for cleansing the peristomal skin when no water is available. It should be remembered that many public lavatories have the wash basin and water supply separate to the toilet cubicle. Similar sachets are also available impregnated with skin protective film. These products help ensure that the emergency kit is small and discreet. Commercial travel kits are available which contain a mirror, bottle for water, scissors and pockets for equipment but many patients make up their own, using an attractive soap bag.

Patients going away on holiday should be advised to calculate their usual appliance use and take considerably more than this away with them. This is because it is always possible that their return may be delayed, or the appliances may be found to be faulty or may need changing more frequently if the weather is hot. It is also advisable for patients to take with them an accurate list of the appliances and accessories they use, including the manufacturer's name and code numbers. The telephone number of a stoma care nurse working near the destination is also helpful.

The accommodation to be used must be carefully selected to ensure that the patient with a stoma has either private bathroom facilities or easy access to a toilet and running water. Many patients opt to rent self-contained accommodation where they have unrestricted use of facilities.

Disposal of used appliances may worry stoma patients away from home. The soiled appliance should be emptied and sealed into a plastic bag, it should then be well wrapped and can then be discarded into a rubbish bin or the 'sani-bin' in the ladies' toilets. Specially designed disposal bags for use when travelling can be purchased. One or two appliance companies supply such bags free of charge to customers.

Foreign travel

Travelling abroad may present some additional problems which need consideration and preparation prior to departure.

Climate

In hot climates the patient will perspire more freely, which may result in water and salt depletion in patients who have an ileostomy. They should thus be advised to drink extra fluids (particularly fruit juice which is rich in potassium) and may need salt replacement tablets. Some appliances are not suitable for use in very hot temperatures as the skin protective and adhesive may melt and compromise security. All appliances should be stored in as cool a place as possible away from direct sunlight.

Food

Local water is often best avoided as it may cause stomach upsets and diarrhoea. Ice and salads which have been washed in water should also be regarded with suspicion. Patients who manage their colostomy by irrigation will usually be well advised to use bottled water. Exotic food can produce an upset in bowel function for all of us and patients who have a stoma should be extra cautious. It is sensible for patients to take some treatment with them in case they develop diarrhoea. Patients with colostomies who use closed bags should also take a supply of drainable bags to cope with this eventuality.

In less developed countries facilities may be primitive and supplies difficult to obtain. This may be particularly a problem to Asian patients who may wish to return to their country of origin.

Diseases such as typhoid and cholera may be prevalent in some countries and patients should seek advice about vaccination prior to travelling.

Insurance

It is wise to be cautious when considering travel insurance and patients should check carefully that pre-existing medical conditions are not excluded. The ostomy associations will advise their members on travel insurance and some have special arrangements for travel insurance that will cover pre-existing conditions.

It is advisable for patients to familiarize themselves with the procedures for obtaining medical treatment or making an insurance claim before setting off. EEC countries have a reciprocal health agreement with the United Kingdom which gives citizens entitlement to emergency medical treatment free of charge. To benefit form E111 must be obtained from the DHSS offices (where an explanatory leaflet SA36 is also available) and completed before the journey.

Customs

Patients are often anxious in case they are asked embarrassing questions if their stoma care supplies are discovered by Customs. A travel certificate is available from the ostomy associations which explains in four languages about the operation and the need to wear appliances. This certificate must be signed by a doctor.

Air travel

Many stoma patients find it quite possible to change their appliances in an aircraft lavatory. Some aircrafts have a shelf which folds down for changing a baby, and this is ideal as a surface to spread equipment on. Soiled bags can be wrapped and put into the facility for sanitary towel disposal.

It is essential that stoma care equipment is split between hand luggage and the main luggage in the aircraft hold to help prevent a panic if luggage goes astray. Many commercial airlines will carry medical supplies in addition to the normal baggage allowance free of charge, provided they are informed when a reservation is made.

Inflammable liquids must not be carried on aeroplanes due to the risk of explosion. If patients use a solvent to clean off adhesive around the stoma they should check that it is non-flammable.

Many patients notice an increase in flatus arising from the changing pressure in the aircraft cabin. This could result in the appliance 'ballooning' and leakage may result. Patients should use a pouch with a flatus filter when travelling by air and should avoid flatus-producing foods and aerated drinks before and during the flight.

The time spent on preparation and planning for a trip away is well rewarded as, once any obstacles have been overcome, the sense of progress and liberation is immense. It is often a positive sign that the patient is regaining his self-confidence if he feels able to travel freely and stay away from home overnight.

REFERENCES

1. Klidjian, A.M. (1981) Problems of nutrition in surgical patients: part 1. *Update*, April Vol.22, No. 7.
2. Kennedy, H.J., Al-Dujailu, E.A.S., Edwards, C.R.W. & Trulove, S.C. (1983) Water and electrolyte balance in subjects with a permanent ileostomy. *Gut, 24*, 702–705.
3. Gazzard, B.G. & Dawson, A.M. (1978) Diets and stomas. *Intestinal Stomas*. Ed. Todd, I. Chap.16, pp.133–149. London: Heinemann.
4. Gazzard, B.G., Saunders, B. & Dawson, A.M. (1978) Diets and stoma function. *British Journal of Surgery, 65*, 642–644.
5. Thomson, T.J., Runce, J. & Khan, A. (1970) The effect of diet on ileostomy functions. *Gut, 11*, 482–485.
6. Bingham, McNeil, & Cummings. (1977) Diet for the ileostomist. *Journal of Human Nutrition, 31*, 365–366.
7. Henley, A. (1980) Practical care of Asian patients. *Nursing, No. 16*, August 683–686.
8. Religions and Cultures: A Guide to Patients Beliefs and Customs for Health Service Staff (1978) Prepared by Lothian Community Relations Council.
9. Aliza, Y. (1984) The influence of Jewish religious laws on orthodox Jewish ostomates in Israel. *Proceedings of World Council of Enterostomal Therapists, 5th Biennial Congress*.
10. Whitethread, M. (1981) Ostomists: a world of difference. *Journal of Community Nursing*, August, 4–6.
11. Parmar, M.D. (1985) Family care and ethnic minorities. *Nursing* (2nd Series), *2, No.36*, 1068–1071.
12. Henley, A. (1979) *Asian Patients in Hospital and At Home*. King Edward's Hospital Fund. Pitman Medical Press.
13. Speck, P. (1976) East comes West. *Nursing Times*, 29 April. 662–664.
14. Davitz, L.J., Sameshima, Y. & Davitz, J. (1976) Suffering as viewed in six different cultures. *American Journal of Nursing, 96*, 1296–1297.
15. Rolstad, B.S., Wilson, G. & Rothengerger, D.A. (1983) Sexual concerns in the patient with an ileostomy. *Diseases of the Colon and Rectum, 26*, 170–171.
16. MacDonald, L.D., Anderson, H.R. & Bennett, A.E. (1982) *Cancer Patients in the Community: Outcome of Care and Quality of Survival in Rectal Cancer*. London: DHSS. June.

17. Devlin, H.B. & Plant, J.A. (1979) Sexual function: an aspect of stoma care. *British Journal of Sexual Medicine, 6*, 33–37.
18. Crown, S. (1981) Sexual problems. In *Going Home: A Guide for Helping Patients on Leaving Hospital*. Ed. Simpson, J.E.P. & Lavill, R. Chap.18, pp.220–232. Churchill Livingstone.
19. Brouillette, J.N., Pryor, E. & Fox, T.A. (1981) Evaluation of sexual dysfunction in the female following rectal resection and intestinal stoma. *Diseases of the Colon and Rectum*, 24, pp.96–102.
20. Snow, B. (1984) Ileostomy, sexual problems and self image. *Nursing*, October 2, No.30.
21. Dlin, B.M., Perlman, A. & Ringold, E. (1969) Psychosexual response to ileostomy and colostomy. *American Journal of Psychiatry, 126*, September. *3*, 374–381.
22. Dlin, B.M. & Perlman, A. (1972) Sex after ileostomy or colostomy. *Medical Aspects of Human Sexuality*, July, 32–43.
23. Devlin, H.B. & Plant, J.A. (1979) Sexual function: an aspect of stoma care—part III. *British Journal of Sexual Medicine, 6*, 22–26.
24. Ainslie, S. (1984) Sexuality and the cancer sufferer. *Nursing Mirror, 159*, (19 September) 38–40.
25. Burnham, W.R., Lennard-Jones, J.E. & Brooke, B.N. (1977) Sexual problems among married ileostomists. *Gut, 18*, 673–677.
26. Daines, B., Holdsworth, A.V. (1982) Impotence. *Nursing Times*, (5 May), 763–765.
27. Snow, B. (1980) Self image and the ostomist. *British Journal of Sexual Medicine*, (June) 7, 44.
28. Young, C.H. (1982) Sexual implications of stoma surgery. *Clinics in Gastroenterology, 11*, 383–391.
29. Willoughby, C.P. (1980) Ulcerative colitis and pregnancy. *Topics in Gastroenterology, 8*, 177–190.
30. Barwin, B.N., Harley, J.M. & Wilson, W. (1985) Ileostomy and pregnancy. *British Journal of Clinical Practice, 28*, (July) 7, 256–258.
31. Devlin, H.B. (1985) *Stoma Care To-day*. Published for the Medicine Publishing Foundation and sponsored by Coloplast Ltd.

17 Hints and tips

Working with stoma patients constantly provides the opportunity to collect together many tips and helpful suggestions that can be passed from one patient to the next. The catalogue of ideas that follows are not all my own, they have been collected from a variety of patients and from my fellow stoma care nurses.

EMPTYING BAGS

Drainable bags

These can be emptied directly into the lavatory—a piece of toilet paper put into the pan helps prevent splashing. Many patients prefer to sit on the lavatory and empty the appliance between their legs rather than bending over.

Closed bags

If about 1 cm is turned up at the bottom of the bag and secured with tape, when the bag is removed this can be released and it provides a clean piece of plastic to cut off allowing the bag to be emptied. The bag can then be either held in the stream of the flushing toilet or hung in the stream using a bent wire coathanger, allowing the water to rinse the bag.

Baby oil or liquid paraffin within the appliance makes it easier to empty cleanly.

LIMITED BATHROOM FACILITIES

If space in the bathroom is limited a plank of wood about 45 cm wide and long enough to put across the bath may be used as a shelf for equipment when the appliance is being changed. When not in use it can be stood out of the way against a wall.

REMOVING APPLIANCE

A skin-protective film often aids removal of the appliance from the skin. If a small area of the adhesive is turned over before the bag is applied this forms a tab to begin removal. Adhesives are often best removed dry, when damp a film of adhesive remains on the skin.

DISPOSAL

A large sheet of newspaper should be spread on the floor or in the bottom of a dry bath so the soiled appliance and other waste can be dropped onto it. This can then be parcelled up before being put into the dustbin. Empty plastic bags (saved from shopping) can also be useful to drop soiled appliances into. Some manufacturers supply these free of charge to their customers.

KEEPING CLOTHES AWAY

To allow both hands to be free to deal with the appliance, clothing can be clipped out of the way with two clothes pegs on a tape hung around the neck (Fig. 60).

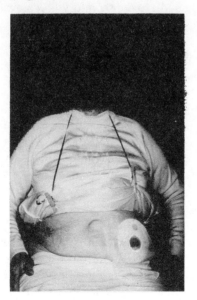

Fig. 60. *Clothing held away from the stoma by clothes pegs.*

CLEANSING

Plain warm water is adequate since soaps can dry the skin and cause irritation. Kitchen paper towels are best for wiping because they do not disintegrate when wet. The skin must be dry prior to putting on an appliance.

It is possible to buy impregnated tissues in a small sachet (Stoma-wipes) for cleansing the peristomal skin, and these are useful when travelling. Ordinary skin-freshener tissues and baby products should be avoided as these may be astringent and dry the skin, or greasy and prevent the appliance sticking.

REMOVING FILLER PASTE

It is preferable to leave a small amount of paste around the stoma than to rub too hard to remove it.

HAIR

Hair beneath an appliance should be cut short or shaved carefully to prevent leakage and avoid discomfort on removal.

SIZE OF APPLIANCE

Gasket/flange size is governed by the size of the stoma and its shape. All the skin around the stoma should be protected from contact with effluent but the stoma must not be nipped. Regular measuring is important to accommodate changes in stoma size.

The size of the bag used is governed by the capacity required and the ability to empty or change the bag regularly.

ODOUR

Odour should only be apparent when the appliance is changed or emptied. If this is particularly offensive a substance within the bag may help, such as vanilla essence (two or three drops), odour absorbing powder, deodorizing fluid, an aspirin tablet or mouth wash concentrate. Handbag-size aerosols of air fresheners are also available for use when away from home.

Offensive urine from a urostomy may be offset by putting a few drops of vinegar into the bag.

STORAGE

Appliances should be stored in a cool place away from direct heat or sunlight, for instance in a spare bedroom. They should also be used in rotation to avoid old stock accumulating.

LEAKAGE

Check size of gasket, and type of appliance. Look for skin creases and delves. (See Chapter 14.)

SORE SKIN

Elicit cause if possible. (See Chapter 14.) Protect from further damage and stripping by applying a skin wafer cut to the exact size of the stoma. Fill gaps and crevices with filler paste; these may sting on the raw areas, and a sprinkle of barrier powder helps to relieve this.

SEVERE SKIN EXCORIATION

This often heals quickly if baby milk powder is mixed into a thin paste and applied to the skin on gauze two-hourly for 24-hours. During this time no appliance is worn. Egg white may also be beneficial as the protein aids healing.

If greasy preparations are applied to the peristomal skin they should be sealed over with an Op-site dressing prior to fitting an appliance.

VACUUM WITHIN BAGS

This may result in leakage or faeces 'pancaking' around the opening into the appliance. A little air should be put into the bag prior to application. If a flatus patch is used which allows the air to escape, a horizontal pleat should be made in the bag. A tissue screwed into a ball and put into the bag prior to application also helps prevent a vacuum occurring. Sticky plastic strips are available to stick onto the outside of the bag; these are then bent to hold the front of the bag away from the stoma. If a flatus patch is not needed it may be occluded with a vinyl patch.

EXCESSIVE FLATUS

This can be due to diet, smoking, swallowing air when eating, missing meals or taking fizzy drinks. Try to identify the cause; omitting possible culprit foods or eating natural yoghurt may help.

TRAVEL

Appliances should be split between hand luggage and suitcases while travelling. Extras should be taken in case of emergency— unexpected delay in return or faulty appliances. Check that the appliance is suitable for hot climates, and store in a cool place, particularly abroad. Bags for disposal are available either to purchase or free from some appliance companies. Carry a list of appliances and accessories with the relevant code numbers.

Obtain a travel certificate for Customs and form E111 for medical services if visiting EEC countries.

Be prepared for stomach upsets—take drainable bags, medication, etc. Ileostomists should also take extra fluids and salt tablets. (See Chapter 16.)

CLIMATE

Some appliances are unsuitable for hot environments. In hot weather keep appliances in the salad drawer of the fridge.

SPORTS AND ACTIVITIES

Many manufacturers produce small appliances or caps. These are ideal for sports, swimming and on intimate occasions as they are very discreet.

SWIMWEAR

Specially designed swimwear is available for purchase by patients with stomas. However, the majority of patients find that ordinary swimwear is much less expensive and perfectly adequate if carefully selected.

Highly patterned fabrics are particularly suitable and many women opt for styles which gather at the front. If an appliance is detectable beneath the sleek lines of a swimsuit then a motif can be sewn in place to detract the eye.

CLOTHING

Although stoma patients should not find it necessary to alter their choice of clothing they may find that purchasing from a mail order catalogue or chain store is advantageous initially as exchanges are welcomed. This provides them with the opportunity to try clothes on in the privacy of their own home where they can ensure that the appliance is not detectable, which is not always possible in a communal changing room.

Patients who like to wear tight-fitting clothes may find it helpful to fit their bag at an angle so that when effluent collects any fullness is accommodated by the hollow in the abdomen above the pubic bone.

BAG COVERS

These help disguise contents within the bag and reduce sweating. They can also act as a morale booster. Patients can make very attractive covers from scraps of fabric, cotton and disposable covers are available on prescription.

If covers slip they can either be secured to the skin with a short length of tape or, if the patient is wearing a belt, they can attach the cover to the belt with a snap fastener.

BABIES

A drainable bag is usually most suitable for babies to prevent stripping the baby's delicate skin by constant removal. A two-piece appliance may be advantageous for a baby weighing more than 5 kg, provided no pressure is applied when fitting. The skin beneath the appliance should be protected with a barrier film. The size of the bag is not as important as ensuring an adequate area of adhesion keeps the appliance secure.

Dungarees and all-in-one suits are helpful as the baby grows in preventing him from interfering with the appliance.

SEAT BELTS

Some stoma patients are reluctant to wear seat belts claiming that they are uncomfortable and cause leakage. If the lap strap sits across the stoma a little extra length of belt can be pulled out and secured at the side with a bulldog paper clip so that it does not tighten. The belt will still hold the patient secure in the seat in cases of emergency. Alternatively, a wedge of foam rubber placed beneath the lap strap to the side of the stoma will help relieve pressure.

Devices designed to avoid discomfort due to seat belts tightening, such as the 'Klunk Klip' are available commercially from car accessory shops.

UROSTOMIES

Phosphate deposits

Infected or alkaline urine may cause white barnacle-like encrustations to form on the stoma. These may be removed by neutralizing them with an acidic substance, for example bathing in a solution of 5% acetic acid or applying Aci-Jel (Ortho-Cilag) is usually successful. High doses of ascorbic acid (4 gm daily) given orally may also help in overcoming these encrustations.

Night drainage

The night drainage tube may be passed down the leg of the pyjamas to prevent kinking. Some types of appliance are designed so that the outlet tap can be closed with the tube in situ, in this case a 15–20 cm length can be left in position so that men can empty the bag via their trouser flies.

Spina bifida patients may keep longer lengths of tubing in situ to put over the toilet while remaining in their wheelchair.

Diabetics

Diabetics with an ileal conduit should not rely upon urine testing to estimate glycosuria as glucose may be reabsorbed from the urine by the ileal loop.

Giving enemas

It is difficult for patients to retain enemas due to the lack of sphincter muscles. Enemas which contain little fluid but are hypertonic are often most suitable.

If an oil retention enema is required then a Foley catheter may be inserted well into the stoma and the balloon inflated with up to 5 ml of water to act as a plug. The oil is then instilled via the catheter and the balloon is left inflated for a few minutes.

If the substance introduced is greasy it may prove difficult to fit an appliance after the instillation. It is helpful to use a two-piece appliance that clips together for this procedure. The flange should be affixed to the skin while it is dry and then a drainable bag clipped in place after the enema is given.

Knowledge of these hints and tips can be most helpful to the nurse when she is coping with the practical aspects of stoma care.

Index

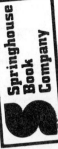
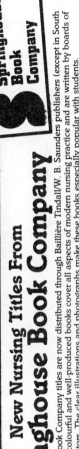

THE CNP SERIES from Baillière Tindall

New nursing techniques are continually being developed to meet the growing complexity of medical care. The **Current Nursing Practice** series is designed to enable the nurse practitioner to study a specialist subject in greater detail. The information is topical, up-to-date and takes a problem-solving approach to nursing care.

titles published to date have received high praise . . . .

A. Stalker
EAR, NOSE AND THROAT NURSING (6/e)

". . . presents ear, nose and throat nursing in an attractive, easily-read format . . . The book is divided into six sections. Among the subjects discussed are the nose and accessory sinuses; the pharynx; larynx; trachea; and oesophagus. These sections are then sub-divided to discuss relevant anatomy and physiology; disorders and disease which may occur; and the medical or surgical treatment necessary. Up-to-date nursing techniques related to the particular structures are approached in a problem-solving manner . . ."
NURSING MIRROR, 30th January 1985

0 7020 1010 3   224pp   100 ills   Pb   1984   Baillière Tindall (UK)

G. Purchese & D. Allan
NEUROMEDICAL AND NEUROSURGICAL NURSING (2/e)

". . . extensively revised . . . extremely well written, clear and concise, providing an up-to-date guide and reference book for both qualified and learner nurses. The first chapter gives an introduction to neurological nursing . . . Chapters two and three are concerned with admission and assessment and investigations; I found the latter particularly informative. Subsequent chapters deal with conditions ranging from epilepsy, infections and raised intracranial pressure to craniotomy – pre- and postoperative care and pain relief. Emphasis in each chapter is placed on the nurse's role in the care of these patients. The final chapter is concerned with the therapeutic team. The book also contains many well labelled drawings . . ."
SENIOR NURSE, 13th March 1985

". . . The publishers are to be congratulated on a well produced book. Clear layout of the text gives welcome clarity to the topic. In particular the excellent diagrams add much and are to be especially commended . . . Overall I can wholeheartedly recommend this book for both RGN students and more specialised neuromedical and neurosurgical students . . ."
JOURNAL OF ADVANCED NURSING, No. 10, 1985

". . . the book is topical, it is comprehensive and clearly written . . ."
NURSING STANDARD, November 1984

". . . I have found it invaluable . . . As a text for neuromedical/neurosurgical nursing I recommend this as essential reading . . ."
NURSING MIRROR, 17th October 1984

0 7020 1030 8   325pp   57 ills   Pb   1984   Baillière Tindall (UK)

J. V. Harvey Kemble & B. E. Lamb
PLASTIC SURGICAL AND BURNS NURSING

"How refreshing to read a book on plastic surgery by English authors, hard to find these days. The book is a pleasure to read, the separation of specific nursing problems is carried out concisely. The concepts of plastic surgery are described clearly in the first three chapters giving the reader a good understanding, before going into specialties, where all aspects of plastic surgery are given good coverage . . . I would recommend this book to anyone interested in plastic surgery . . ."
NURSING STANDARD, August 1984

". . . This book is excellent value and should be bought by all nurses involved with plastic surgery patients. Plastic surgeons could also read it with advantage, as it would give them a valuable insight into the work of their nursing colleagues."
BRITISH BOOK NEWS, November 1984

0 7020 1029 4   397pp   110 ills   Pb   1984   Baillière Tindall (UK)

D. Bradley
ACCIDENT AND EMERGENCY NURSING (2/e)

". . . This title, which has undergone major revision, provides information and skills for both learners and trained staff. Covers all types of emergency, as well as major and minor trauma. Photographs and drawings, which are very clear, are enormously helpful."
JOURNAL OF THE INSTITUTE OF HEALTH EDUCATION, Vol. 22, No. 3

0 7020 1048 0   352pp   180 ills   Pb   1984   Baillière Tindall (UK)

and new . . .

J. Huskisson
APPLIED DIETETICS AND NUTRITION (2/e)

This new edition puts great emphasis on nursing considerations and the role of the nurse as part of the dietary therapeutic team. New chapters have been incorporated on the role of the nurse, haematological disorders, and transitional diets.

0 7020 1101 0   256pp   27 ills   Pb   September 1985   Baillière Tindall (UK)

NEW BOOKS IN THE NAS SERIES
from **Baillière Tindall**

The reliable and well-known NAS series has been redesigned and updated to take account of recent advances in nursing practice and of the introduction of the nursing process.

─ New publications in the NAS series include: ──────────

A. M. F. Storrs
GERIATRIC NURSING (3/e)
"This third edition of Alison Storrs' already popular book represents a welcome update of what has proved to be a useful introduction to geriatric nursing ... The book is extremely informative, very readable and a useful addition to every nursing library. I found it particularly pleasing to see the Scandinavian approach to continuing care being acknowledged and recommended ..."
NURSING MIRROR, 29th May 1985

0 7020 1059 6   208pp   Ills   Pb   1985   Baillière Tindall (UK)

M. Wilson
SURGICAL NURSING (11/e)
"The eleventh edition of this well-known book has been completely rewritten to include: The principles of surgical nursing; common surgical problems and nursing responses; a surgical model based on patients' needs; clear, informative illustrations; and useful suggestions for further reading. The author aims to help nurses plan their individualised care more effectively by using a systematic problem-oriented approach to the care of each type of surgical patient. Each chapter covers a different type of surgery physiologically, then goes on to describe preoperative investigations, types of surgery, related pre- and postoperative nursing activities, aims of nursing care, continuing care and future health considerations ... an invaluable learning and revision aid ..."
NURSING MIRROR, 8th May 1985

0 7020 1061 8   208pp   54 ills   Pb   1985   Baillière Tindall (UK)

G. M. Newton & C. Andrews
MEDICAL NURSING (10/e)
"This small-format paperback is well laid out and lives up to its claim that the information is concise and easily retrieved ..."
SENIOR NURSE, June 1985

"... extensively updated and revised by two new authors who have adopted a problem solving approach to individualised patient care ... the book sets out to be a concise reference which forms the basis of information that nurses require about medical nursing and as such I feel it achieves its aim admirably ..."
NURSING TIMES, 30th January 1985

"Ten successful editions prove the popularity and value of this little book. Using a problem solving approach, it covers the central topics on Medical Nursing, including both the patients and the nursing view points, emphasising from the outset that patients are people first and foremost. Excellent value."
JOURNAL OF THE INSTITUTE OF HEALTH EDUCATION, Vol. 22, No. 3

0 7020 0963 6   288pp   57 ills   Pb   1984   Baillière Tindall (UK)

A. Altschul & M McGovern
PSYCHIATRIC NURSING (6/e)
The sixth edition of this best selling introductory book for students of psychiatric nursing has been revised and rearranged to reflect developments in this specialised field. New material includes the development of the role of the community psychiatric nurse and the nursing implications of the increasing number of elderly patients with organic mental disease. The text offers detailed information on: drug therapy; electroconvulsive therapy; classification of mental disorders; and the legislation related to the Mental Health Acts 1983–1984.

"Like Napoleon's observation that there is a baton in every soldier's knapsack, there must now be an 'Annie Altschul' in every nurse's pocket ... This book should be in every nursing library and on every nurse's bookshelf ... very readable, compassionate and realistic ..."
NURSING MIRROR (from a review of the previous edition)

0 7020 1060 X   368pp   Pb   1985   Baillière Tindall (UK)

D. Thompson & G. Bowman
MEDICAL INVESTIGATIONS
This new title enables the nurse to understand the increasing complexity of medical investigations and the related nursing care. Frequently patients find investigative procedures a greater source of stress and discomfort than the treatment for the illness. This book provides the nurse with the background information needed to skilfully give the appropriate explanations, preparatory and follow-up care. The principles of nursing care are discussed and this includes the moral, ethical and legal considerations. A systems approach is taken to: common medical investigations; possible complications and related nursing care. This new title offers: detailed explanations of investigations; essential information for the nurse's theoretical work; an understanding of the procedures enabling the nurse to reassure patients and minimize their discomfort; and guidance on appropriate nursing responses. This welcome addition to the new format NAS series will be a valuable reference on the ward and in the community.

0 7020 1088 X   224pp   Ills   Pb   1985   Baillière Tindall (UK)

NURSING DICTIONARIES
INVALUABLE AIDS FOR THE NURSING PROFESSION TODAY!

┌─BAILLIÈRE'S DESK TOP LIBRARY─

K. Kasner & D. H. Tindall
Baillière's Nurses' Dictionary (20/e)

For its twentieth edition this well-known dictionary has been radically revised and enlarged with excellent new illustrations. The dictionary includes, for the first time, a number of terms used by the paramedical professions of physiotherapy, radiography and speech therapy.

0 7020 1035 9   328pp   108 ills   Pb
0 7020 1046 4   328pp   108 ills   Hb
1984   Baillière Tindall (UK)

D. Middleton
Baillière's Ward Information (14/e)

This is a thorough revision and update of the factual and essential information required for the ward. It covers a wide range of day-to-day problems from ward emergencies to normal biochemical values. A book for every busy nurse to carry in her pocket.

0 7020 1032 4   213pp   Ills   Pb
1984   Baillière Tindall (UK)

E. B. Steen
Baillière's Abbreviations in Medicine (5/e)

This handy-sized dictionary has once again been updated and enlarged. It lists more than 15,000 common medical and related abbreviations. New information is included on databases and the useful appendixes list the abbreviations for major journals, and include a guide to other reference books.

0 7020 1036 7   224pp   Pb
1984   Baillière Tindall (UK)

M. Adams
Baillière's Midwives' Dictionary (7/e)

This edition represents the most extensive revision of the dictionary since its original publication in 1951. The revisions reflect the changes of the last five years, including the formation of the UK Central Council, and the introduction of new laws and legislation on midwifery, obstetrics and nursing.

0 7020 0931 8   368pp   83 ills   Pb
1983   Baillière Tindall (UK)

Baillière's Desk Top Libary   0 7020 1055 3
4 titles as listed above   Slipcased
1984   Baillière Tindall (UK)

┌─also recommended . . .─

D-E. Chabner
The Language of Medicine (3/e)

This new edition has been meticulously reviewed and updated to include the latest terminology and a 'Practical Applications' section.

0 7216 1184 2   730pp   Ills   Pb
March 1985   W. B. Saunders

D. Duff & J. M. Aylward
A Metric Guide for Health Professionals on Dosages and Solutions

This is a workbook on metric calculations for all health professionals. All units are in SI, and included in the book are pre-test and post-test questions and answers.

0 7216 1453 1   ca 190pp   Ills   PbSp
January 1985   W. B. Saunders (Canada)

S. B. Sloane
Medical Abbreviations and Eponyms

This book offers a comprehensive listing of medical abbreviations, acronyms, symbols and eponyms for anyone involved directly or indirectly with medical records.

0 7216 1522 8   ca 432pp   Pb
July 1985   W. B. Saunders

P. Leonard
Building A Medical Vocabulary

This self-paced medical terminology text approaches vocabulary building with a new innovative style providing the basics (roots, prefixes and suffixes) as well as fundamentals, to help students interpret the meaning of new words.

0 7216 1051 X   350pp   30 ills   PbSp
1983   W. B. Saunders

B. F. Miller & C. B. Keane
Encyclopaedia and Dictionary of Medicine, Nursing and Allied Health (3/e)

0 7216 6363 X   Indexed (Deluxe) Version
Durable Flex Binding
0 7216 6364 8   Plain (Economy) Version   Pb
1270 pp   185 ills   1983   W. B. Saunders

Dorland
Dorland's Pocket Medical Dictionary (23/e)

0 7216 3166 5   Indexed Version
0 7216 3167 3   Non-Index Version
840pp   Ills (16 Col. plates)   flexible cover
1982   W. B. Saunders